Praise for *Mastering Ph*

MW00353044

"The authors have an exceptional ability to make genetics and genomics accessible to nurses, and this text on pharmacogenomics is no exception. Nurses in every setting will find applications to their own work."

–Heather Skirton, PhD, RGN, RGC
Professor of Applied Health Genetics, Plymouth University (UK)
Chair of the European Board of Medical Genetics

"This book is an essential resource for healthcare providers as we fast-forward to affordable gene sequencing for identifying, understanding, and treating individuals based on the merger/convergence of therapeutic treatment and personalized genetic information. This is critical reading for those already practicing and teaching and required reading for those preparing to launch their careers as professional clinicians."

–Annette Wysocki, PhD, RN, FAAN
Associate Dean for Research and Professor, University of Massachusetts Amherst
Former Scientific Director of National Institute of Nursing Research (NINR) and
Project Manager of the Summer Genetics Institute at NINR

"*Mastering Pharmacogenomics: A Nurse's Handbook for Success* is an excellent resource explaining the fundamentals of tailored medicine. The strength of the book is in the clarity with which complex concepts are presented, aided by features such as nurse-centered case examples and end-of-chapter summaries. This book is an easy-to-read, accessible volume, making it a "must have" for the library of every level of nurse, from student to advanced practice."

–Bernice Coleman, PhD, ACNP
Nurse Scientist, Nurse Practitioner, Heart Transplantation, Mechanical Assist Device Programs
Nursing Education and Heart Institute, Cedars-Sinai Medical Center

"We are at a point in time where we have a critical mass of knowledge about the effect of genomic variability on health. Current and future healthcare providers need to have a basic understanding of pharmacogenomics and be able to use this information to inform practice and communicate with patients. *Mastering Pharmacogenomics: A Nurse's Handbook for Success* covers the basic science content needed to understand the current science of pharmacogenomics but has the added value of providing real-life applicability of crucial concepts. The book is extremely well organized, discusses important pharmacogenomics concepts within specific populations, addresses key ethical considerations, and provides online resources that will help to keep the content current for the reader. Educators of future healthcare providers, current healthcare providers, and students will all benefit from gaining an understanding of pharmacogenomics through the patient-centered approach used in *Mastering Pharmacogenomics: A Nurse's Handbook for Success.*"

–Yvette P. Conley, PhD
Professor of Nursing and Human Genetics, University of Pittsburgh

"Authored by experts in their field, this book provides a wealth of current and well-referenced pharmacogenomics material. It will be invaluable to the growing number of healthcare courses requiring students to study genomics. Readers are provided with a text covering the necessary biological framework. However, the uniqueness of this book is that it retains its practice focus on real-world healthcare applications."

–Caroline Benjamin, PhD, RGN, RGC
Guild Research Fellow–Health, HeRMI (Health Research Methodology and Implementation Hub)
UK Registered Genetic Counsellor
Hon. Research Fellow I Liverpool Women's NHS Foundation Trust

Mastering Pharmacogenomics

A Nurse's Handbook for Success

Dale Halsey Lea, MPH, RN, CGC, APNG; Dennis J. Cheek, PhD, RN, FAHA;
Daniel Brazeau, PhD; Gayle Brazeau, PhD

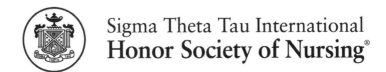

Sigma Theta Tau International
Honor Society of Nursing®

The Honor Society of Nursing, Sigma Theta Tau International (STTI) is a nonprofit organization whose mission is to support the learning, knowledge, and professional development of nurses committed to making a difference in health worldwide. Founded in 1922, STTI has 130,000 members in 86 countries. Members include practicing nurses, instructors, researchers, policymakers, entrepreneurs and others. STTI's 499 chapters are located at 695 institutions of higher education throughout Australia, Botswana, Brazil, Canada, Colombia, Ghana, Hong Kong, Japan, Kenya, Malawi, Mexico, the Netherlands, Pakistan, Portugal, Singapore, South Africa, South Korea, Swaziland, Sweden, Taiwan, Tanzania, United Kingdom, United States, and Wales. More information about STTI can be found online at www.nursingsociety.org.

Sigma Theta Tau International
550 West North Street
Indianapolis, IN, USA 46202

To order additional books, buy in bulk, or order for corporate use, contact Nursing Knowledge International at 888.NKI.4YOU (888.654.4968/US and Canada) or +1.317.634.8171 (outside US and Canada).

To request a review copy for course adoption, email solutions@nursingknowledge.org or call 888.NKI.4YOU (888.654.4968/US and Canada) or +1.317.634.8171 (outside US and Canada).

To request author information, or for speaker or other media requests, contact Marketing, Honor Society of Nursing, Sigma Theta Tau International at 888.634.7575 (US and Canada) or +1.317.634.8171 (outside US and Canada).

ISBN: 9781938835704

EPUB ISBN: 9781938835711

PDF ISBN: 9781938835728

MOBI ISBN: 9781938835735

Library of Congress Cataloging-in-Publication Data

Lea, Dale Halsey, author.
  Mastering pharmacogenomics : a nurse's handbook for success / Dale Halsey Lea, Dennis J. Cheek, Daniel Brazeau, Gayle Brazeau.
    p. ; cm.
  Includes bibliographical references.
  ISBN 978-1-938835-70-4 (print : alk. paper) -- ISBN 978-1-938835-71-1 (Epub) -- ISBN 978-1-938835-72-8 (PDF) -- ISBN 978-1-938835-73-5 (Mobi)
  I. Cheek, Dennis J., author. II. Brazeau, Daniel A., author. III. Brazeau, Gayle A., author. IV. Sigma Theta Tau International, issuing body. V. Title.
  [DNLM: 1. Drug Therapy--nursing. 2. Pharmacogenetics. WY 100.1]
  RM301.3.G45
  615.1'9--dc23
                    2014042045

First Printing, 2015

Publisher: Dustin Sullivan
Acquisitions Editor: Emily Hatch
Editorial Coordinator: Paula Jeffers
Cover Designer: Michael Tanamachi
Interior Design/Page Layout: Rebecca Batchelor
Illustrator: Clint Lahnen

Principal Book Editor: Carla Hall
Development and Project Editor: Brian Walls
Copy Editor: Teresa Artman
Proofreader: Barbara Bennett
Indexer: Cheryl Jackson Lenser

Dedication

We dedicate *Mastering Pharmacogenomics: A Nurse's Handbook for Success* to all nurses worldwide.

Acknowledgments

We would like to acknowledge the International Society of Nurses in Genetics (ISONG) for its significant role in fostering the professional growth of nurses in genetics and genomics around the world. We would like to acknowledge Kathleen Calzone, PhD, RN, APNG, FAAN, who is a significant, inspiring national leader in nursing genetics/genomics. Finally, we would like to also acknowledge Sigma Theta Tau International (STTI) for its support of this project. Thank you.

About the Authors

Dale Halsey Lea, MPH, RN, CGC, APNG

Dale Halsey Lea is an advanced practice nurse in genetics and a board certified genetic counselor. Lea has worked for more than 30 years in the field of genetics. From 1983 to 2005, she worked as a genetic counselor in a public health genetics clinic in Maine. From 2005 to 2010, she worked as a health educator for the National Human Genome Research Institute in both the Education and Community Involvement Branch and the Genomic Healthcare Branch. In her position as health educator, Lea oversaw genetics and genomics educational projects and resources that reached out to the general public and healthcare providers. In the fall of 2010, Lea began a consulting position with the Maine State Genetics Program, where she has worked with the program to develop a Maine State Genetics Plan. Lea has published widely in the nursing literature on genetic and genomic topics. She has also taught an online genetics and genomics course for nurses. She has written textbooks on genetics and genomics for nurses and has given genetics/genomics presentations to nurses worldwide. Lea received a baccalaureate degree in English from Wheaton College in 1972. She received an associate degree in nursing from Marymount College of Virginia School of Nursing in 1978, and her baccalaureate degree in nursing from Westbrook College/University of New England School of Nursing in 1988, graduating with high honors. She then went on to get a master's degree in public health education and health promotion from Loma Linda University in 1992. She has been a member of the International Society of Nurses in Genetics (ISONG) since 1986 and was a founding member and former president. She was also a fellow of the American Academy of Nursing.

Dennis J. Cheek, PhD, RN, FAHA

Dennis J. Cheek is the Abell-Hanger Professor in Gerontological Nursing at Texas Christian University-Harris College of Nursing and Health Sciences, with a joint appointment in the School of Nurse Anesthesia. He received his bachelor of science in nursing from California State University, Fresno and his master of science in nursing from the University of California, San Francisco with a focus in critical care nursing and education. He received his doctor of philosophy in cellular and molecular pharmacology and physiology from the University of Nevada, Reno and was awarded a Nevada AHA Affiliate Post-Doctoral Fellowship to continue his research. His teaching responsibilities include undergraduate pharmacology, graduate pathophysiology and pharmacology, nurse anesthesia pharmacology, and cardiovascular physiology, as well as one of the core courses in the new Doctor of nursing practice program at TCU. Along with his teaching responsibilities, he is continuing his program of research in the established Nursing Research Laboratory, studying the effects of age and exercise on vascular endothelial cells. Cheek has been a member of the Council on Cardiovascular Nursing since 2000 and was inducted as a fellow of the American Heart Association (FAHA). He has published in numerous journals, including *American Journal of Critical Care, American Association of Critical-Care Nurses Clinical Issues, AANA Journal, Biological Research in Nursing, Circulation Research, Critical Care Nurse, Heart & Lung, International Journal of Sports Medicine, Journal of Aging Research, Journal of Emergency Nursing, Medicine & Science in Sports & Exercise, The Journal of Cardiovascular Nursing,* and *Proceedings of the National Academy of Sciences.*

Daniel Brazeau, PhD

Daniel Brazeau is director of the University of New England's Genomics, Analytics and Proteomics Core (GAPc) and a research associate professor in the Department of Pharmaceutical Sciences, College of Pharmacy. The GAPc is a research training facility providing expertise, technologies, and most importantly, training support for faculty and students. He received his BS and MS in biology from the University of Toledo and earned his PhD in biological sciences (1989) from the University at Buffalo. After completing postdoctoral training in population genetics at the University of Houston, he was a research assistant professor in the Department of Zoology at the University of Florida and director of the University of Florida's Genetic Analysis Laboratory in the Interdisciplinary Research Center for Biotechnology. For 10 years prior to joining UNE, he was a research associate professor in the Department of Pharmaceutical Sciences at the University at Buffalo and director of the University at Buffalo's Pharmaceutical Genetics Laboratory. Brazeau's research interests involve the areas of population molecular genetics and genomics. He teaches courses in molecular genetics methodologies and a required course in pharmacogenomics for graduate and pharmacy professional students. Brazeau is also a participating scientist in the National Science Foundation's Geneticist-Educator Network Alliances (GENA), working with high school science teachers to incorporate genetics into the classroom. He has served as chair of the Biological Sciences section in 2008 and is one of the founding chairs of the new Pharmacogenomics Special Interest Group in the American Association of Colleges of Pharmacy.

Gayle Brazeau, PhD

Gayle Brazeau is currently dean and professor in the College of Pharmacy at the University of New England. She received a BS in pharmacy and an MS in pharmaceutical sciences from the University of Toledo in 1980 and 1983, respectively. She received a PhD in pharmaceutics from the University at Buffalo, State University of New York in 1989. Previously, she was a faculty member at the University of Houston, the University of Florida, and the University at Buffalo. Brazeau is an associate editor for the *American Journal of Pharmaceutical Education* and serves on several editorial advisory boards for other scientific journals. She has served as an elected officer, committee member, and committee chair for numerous scientific and professional organizations, including chair of the Council of Faculties and Council of Deans for AACP and chair of the Student and Post-Doc Outreach and Development Committee for AAPS. She has been the recipient of teaching and student recognition awards at the University at Buffalo, University of Florida, and University of Houston. She served as a member or chair on FDA, USP, and SBIR/STTR NIH panels and committees. Her pedagogical research interests focus on curricular and course assessment strategies, design, and assessment of student learning. Her laboratory research interests focus on investigating the biochemical and toxicological interactions of drugs or excipients with skeletal muscle following intramuscular or systemic administration and the role of myostatin in muscle-wasting conditions. Other research interests include the development of intramuscular formulations with reduced muscle damage upon injection without altering drug bioavailability and the importance of pharmacogenomics in contemporary patient care. She is the author or coauthor of more than 50 peer-reviewed papers, chapters, books, and other types of publications. She is a recipient of the State University of New York Chancellor's Award for Excellence in Faculty Service. She was a member of the 2005–2006 AACP Academic Leadership Fellows Program and is a member of the Community Health Foundation of Western and Central New York Fellows Action Network. She was recently recognized as a Class of "2013 Nexters" from MaineBiz, which identifies individuals helping to shape growth in the State of Maine.

Contributing Authors

Lisa Bashore, PhD, APRN, CPNP-PC, CPON

Lisa Bashore is currently assistant professor at Texas Christian University (TCU) in the doctor of nursing practice and master's in nursing program. As part of her role, Bashore is support faculty in the advanced pharmacology course. She also is a part-time clinical advanced practice nurse at Cook Children's Medical Center, where she conducts her clinical research and supports the advancement of the survivorship program. She has published several manuscripts on the topics of quality of life, health behaviors, transition practices, and chronic health problems in childhood cancer survivorship. Bashore has more than 20 years of clinical experience in pediatric and adolescent medicine, and has published her research in peer-reviewed journals.

Matthew D'Angelo, DNP, CRNA

Matthew D'Angelo is an assistant professor in the Graduate School of Nursing and serves as the assistant program director of the Nurse Anesthesia Program. D'Angelo has more than 20 years of experience with the U.S. Army Reserve. He enlisted in the Army in 1992 and served as an infantryman. During that time, D'Angelo completed a bachelor of science degree in nursing from the University of Maryland, Baltimore. D'Angelo began his nursing career as a pediatric critical care nurse at the University of Maryland Medical Center. He commissioned as a second lieutenant in the U.S. Army Reserve in 1999. He continued his education and completed a master of science from Georgetown University in 2001. He became a certified registered nurse anesthetist in 2002 and maintained clinical practice at the R. Adams Cowley Shock Trauma Center for nearly a decade. In 2008, D'Angelo completed a doctor of nursing practice degree with an emphasis in fluid resuscitation from the University of Maryland School of Nursing. He has funded research evaluating methods to quantify intravascular volume and its utilization in perioperative fluid administration. D'Angelo has served as a staff nurse anesthetist at the R. Adams Cowley Shock Trauma Center in Baltimore, the University of Maryland Medical Center, Johns Hopkins University, and at The Northwest Hospital Center. In addition to his clinical experiences, D'Angelo has served as the assistant program director for the University of Maryland Nurse Anesthesia Program and has been a clinical preceptor for a variety of nurse anesthesia programs throughout the Baltimore-Washington region. He is a veteran of Operation Iraqi Freedom, having served as the assistant chief of anesthesia nursing for the 345th Combat Support

Hospital located in Al Asad, Iraq. D'Angelo is currently a reviewer for the *American Association of Nurse Anesthetists Journal* (*AANA Journal*) and an onsite reviewer for The Council on Accreditation of Nurse Anesthesia Educational Programs (COA).

Ellen Giarelli, EdD, RN, CRNP

Giarelli is an advanced practice nurse with a postdoctorate degree in psychosocial oncology and HIV/AIDS from the University of Pennsylvania. She is associate professor in the doctoral nursing program at Drexel University College of Nursing and Health Professions. She has an adjunct appointment at the University of Pennsylvania School of Nursing, and is an external advisor and peer reviewer for the UPENN Center for the Integration of Genetic Health Technology (CIGHT). She is president of the International Society of Nurses in Genetics (ISONG).

Giarelli has more than 15 years of experience doing research on the lifelong medical, psychological, social, and healthcare needs of people with genetic disorders diagnosed in childhood that require lifelong, enhanced surveillance and self-management. Study populations include individuals with Marfan syndrome, cancer syndromes such as familial adenomatous polyposis (FAP), multiple endocrine neoplasia type 2a (MEN2s), and autism spectrum disorder (ASD).

She is editor of the book *Nursing of Autism Spectrum Disorder: Evidence-based Integrated Care across the Lifespan* (Springer, 2012), which addresses nursing care of people with ASD by examination of professional nursing skills applied to the specific problems arising from the delivery of healthcare to people with ASD.

Lynnette Howington, DNP, RNC, WHNP-BC, CNL

Lynnette L. Howington is a women's health nurse practitioner and an assistant professor of professional practice at Texas Christian University (TCU). She received her doctorate of nursing practice and bachelor of science in nursing at Texas Christian University and her master of science in nursing at Old Dominion University. She was inducted into Sigma Theta Tau International during her undergraduate work. Howington began teaching at TCU in 2007. While at TCU, she developed (and continues to teach) the genetics course for undergraduate nursing students. Howington has been a maternity nurse for 20 years and a nurse practitioner for 11 years. As a result of this experience, she is part of the teaching team for the women's health/maternity course. Howington is a member of the International Society of Nurses in Genetics

(ISONG) and has given presentations regarding incorporating genetics information into the undergraduate curriculum. As a nurse practitioner, she continues to see patients on a regular basis.

Michelle Munroe, DNP, CNM

Michelle Munroe earned her bachelor of science and master of science in nursing degrees from the University of Maryland at Baltimore and her doctor of nursing practice (DNP) degree from Frontier University. Munroe is a certified nurse midwife who has been continuously practicing for 11 years. As a nurse midwife, she has provided direct care to pregnant women and their families, deployed in support of Operation Iraqi Freedom, and was the chief of the OB/GYN clinic and chief of the midwifery service at Madigan Army Medical Center in Takoma, Washington. She was the chief nurse at Ft. Lee, Virginia, and is currently the assistant dean for student affairs in the Graduate School of Nursing at the Uniformed Services University of the Health Sciences in Bethesda, Maryland. Since arriving at the university, she has had an increased interest in genomics in women's healthcare.

Erika Santos, PhD, RN, MSc

Erika Santos is a nurse with expertise in oncology. She lives in Sao Paulo, Brazil, and in the past 16 years has worked in oncology, focused on hereditary cancer. She is scientific advisor at Hospital Sírio-Libanês, Sao Paulo and coordinator of the Hereditary Cancer Registry. She has a PhD in oncology, is a supervisor at Hospital A.C. Camargo Cancer Graduation Program, and also teaches oncology nursing. She is an active member of International Society of Nurses in Genetics, has sat on the Communication Committee, and has been the editor of the ISONG newsletter since 2007. She has been an ONS member since 2001.

Silvia Regina Secoli, PhD, RN, MSc

Silvia Regina Secoli holds degrees in nursing and a master's in pharmacology at the Faculty of Medical Sciences, UNICAMP and a PhD in nursing at the University of Sao Paulo, Brazil. She is a postdoctoral fellow in pharmacoepidemiology at the Catalan Institute of Pharmacology at the Universitat Autonoma de Barcelona. She is currently associate professor at the School of Nursing, University of Sao Paulo. She has experience in nursing, with emphasis on medical-surgical nursing related to use of drugs, pharmacology, drug interactions, and evaluation of health technologies. She is also a researcher at the Technology Assessment in Health Research Group and the Pharmacoepidemiology Group, both registered in the National Council for Scientific and Technological Development (CNPq).

Diane Seibert, PhD, ARNP, FAANP, FAAN

Seibert is a professor and chair/director of the Family Nurse Practitioner program at the Uniformed Services University in Bethesda, Maryland. She is certified in both women's health and adult nurse practitioner specialties and maintains an active clinical practice at the National Naval Medical Center in Bethesda. Seibert has published and presented widely in the areas of women's health and genetics and is involved in several national task forces and committees working toward improving the genetics competency of the nursing workforce across all practice settings. She leads a multidisciplinary team in the development of an open access, online genetics resource called GeneFacts, which provides rapid and accurate genetic information at the point of care. Seibert received her BSN from Kent State University, her master's degree from the University of Maryland at Baltimore, and her PhD from the University of Maryland at College Park.

Heidi Trinkman, PharmD

Heidi Trinkman is currently the pediatric clinical pharmacy specialist for the hematology/oncology and stem cell transplant program at Cook Children's Medical Center in Fort Worth, Texas. Trinkman is a preceptor for the Cook Children's pharmacy residency program and has been an invited speaker at national meetings. She is active in research and has published in peer-reviewed journals. Trinkman has been practicing in the field of pediatric hematology/oncology pharmacy for 13 years.

John Twomey, PhD, PNP, FNP

John Twomey has been a practicing nurse practitioner for more than 30 years. He retired as a professor of nursing at the MGH Institute of Health Professions in 2013. He completed the Summer Genetics Institute at the National Institute of Nursing in 2001 and was also a postdoctoral fellow in psychosocial genetics at the University of Iowa College of Nursing from 2004–2006. Twomey's doctoral degree is in bioethics, and for the past 15 years, he has studied and written extensively on the bioethical issues inherent in genomic health, particularly family decision-making about genetic testing. He wishes to acknowledge the University of Massachusetts, Boston College of Nursing and Health Sciences for its support of his research for this chapter.

Chris Winkelman, PhD, RN, CCRN, ACNP, CNE, FCCM

Chris Winkelman attended the NIH/NINR Summer Institute, where he developed an interest in the inflammatory cascade. His 10-year program of research examines positioning and activity among chronically, critically ill adults and includes evaluation of serum biomarkers for inflammation, which is a common pathological phenomena in critically ill adults. The biomarkers include interleukins (IL) 6, 8, 10, and 15, IL-1 and IL-1 receptor antagonist, tumor necrosis factor alpha. Several of these molecular messengers have drugs that specifically target their actions and reduce pathology in pro-inflammatory conditions. Pharmacogenomics has been useful in building knowledge about these drug targets. Winkelman has extensive clinical experience in the care of critically ill adults and is certified as both a critical care nurse and an acute care nurse practitioner. As a full-time educator, Winkelman teaches advanced pharmacology to MSN students and directs the Adult-Gerontology Acute Care Nurse program at Case Western Reserve University, The Francis Payne Bolton School of Nursing. He is very grateful to all the patients and students who teach him about preferences and values important to drug selection.

Table of Contents

1   Basics of Genetics and Genomics. 1

Dale Halsey Lea, MPH, RN, CGC, APNG
Chris Winkelman, PhD, RN, CCRN, ACNP, CNE, FCCM

2   Genomic Technologies and Resources. 23

Daniel Brazeau, PhD

3   Basics of Pharmacogenetics 35

Daniel Brazeau, PhD

Foreword

This is a pivotal time in clinical care with the opportunity to use information learned about the contributions of the human genome to health, disease, and response to interventions. However, without the foundational knowledge of the basic principles of human genetics and genomics, nurses will ineffectively apply such information to optimize patient care. Plus, the constant emergence of potential applications of new knowledge necessitates an ongoing quest to maintain currency of the literature to be able to translate such research advances. Such important information for both nursing students and practitioners is provided in *Mastering Pharmacogenomics: A Nurse's Handbook for Success*!

Professionally, I came to recognize the significance of nurses understanding the benefits and risks of applying this foundational genetic and genomic knowledge when I was provided the opportunity by Dr. Francis Collins for an internship at the National Human Genome Research Institute (NHGRI), National Institutes of Health. I came to realize that improved awareness of structure, function, and interactions of the human genome with external influences has the potential to augment options for care. It was during that time that I met a network of nurses within the International Society of Nurses in Genetics (ISONG), including one of this book's authors, Dale Lea. She and I collaborated on writing a couple of textbooks and worked together at the NHGRI. Another ISONG colleague, Dr. Kathleen Calzone, and I established recommended Competencies and Curricula Guidelines with guidance from a consensus panel of nurses. These guidelines are provided as a framework for genomic nursing competency in Chapter 1. A specific core competency of importance for this text focuses on knowledge of pharmacogenetics and pharmacogenomics as essential to all healthcare professionals and an essential component of basic and advanced nursing education and practice. Chapter 4 expands on this and other recommended competency domains and performance indicators, discussing implications for nurses.

This book also provides excellent examples of clinical applications that illustrate challenges nurses face when trying to integrate genomics into healthcare. Chapters offer targeted content of value for nurses working with diverse populations or in specialty settings, providing specifics about the relevance of pharmacogenomics to practice. Resources to assist in facing this challenge are also described, such as interprofessional colleagues (see Chapter 10). I have had the pleasure of partnering with interprofessional colleagues as part of my work within the NHGRI Genomic Healthcare Branch. Colleagues, including pharmacists, physicians, and genetic counselors, all expressed the need to be able to easily access human genetics and genomics resources and collaborated to develop education repositories of value for diverse healthcare providers (i.e., G2C2 http://g-2-c-2.org// and G3C http://g-3-c.org/). Such collaborations of interprofessional colleagues help strengthen the abilities of all healthcare providers to optimize drug therapy and improve patient care.

Why is this information so important for patient care now? I speak from personal experience of the value of using genomic information known about individuals as part of their clinical diagnostic and therapeutic decision-making. When I was diagnosed with cancer in 2001, genetic information was used to maximize my treatment options based on identification of the molecular fingerprints of my lymphoma. I received a targeted therapy that resulted in positive health outcomes, as I am alive and well 13 years later. Plus, advances made since that time have expanded the availability of additional targeted cancer drugs to treat relapsed lymphoma (which I hope I won't ever need), described in Chapter 8. When others say that more research is needed to verify the value of this information before integration into practice, I appreciate their hesitancy. Understanding this complex science requires a commitment to learning more and being able to interpret it in a meaningful way so that positive outcomes can transpire. However, as you can already see, there are possibilities of improved patient outcomes *now*. Because information is already known about the contributions of human genome variation across the continuum of care, you have the prospect of being able to learn more about those possibilities and make a difference for your patients now.

I congratulate you on recognizing the value of learning more about your role in translating pharmacogenomics to make a continuing difference for others. This book will help you begin this ongoing quest to understand the implications of pharmacogenomics for education, practice, research, and policy. Thank you for being innovative and for seeing the importance of your part in preparing patients and their families to have realistic expectations and to improve their ability to make informed decisions about whatever confronts them along their clinical journey.

–Jean Jenkins, PhD, RN, FAAN
Clinical Advisor
Genomic Healthcare Branch
Division of Policy, Communication, and Education
National Human Genome Research Institute, NIH

Introduction

"By the year 2020, gene-based designer drugs are likely to be available for conditions like diabetes, Alzheimer's disease, hypertension, and many other disorders; cancer treatment will precisely target the molecular fingerprints of particular tumors; genetic information will be used routinely to give patients appropriate drug therapy; and the diagnosis and treatment of mental illness will be transformed. By the year 2030, I predict that comprehensive, genomics-based health care will become the norm, with individualized preventive medicine and early detection of illnesses by molecular surveillance; gene therapy and gene-based therapy will be available for many diseases."

–Dr. Francis S. Collins, Director of the National Institute of
Health (http://www.genome.gov/10003482)

The field of genomics and the technologies driving the genomics revolution are rapidly changing the nature of medicine and healthcare. Genomic technologies, and the information amassed from the studies now made possible with these technologies, bring within reach the ultimate goal of understanding the nature of human disease and how best to treat or avoid much human suffering. In fact, genomics has become integral to all fields in the life sciences. In the post-genomic years, patient care and the drugs and diagnostics drawn upon to treat patients will be determined by specific molecular targets underlying disease subtypes. This individualization of disease will make possible far more specific, and hopefully successful, therapeutic interventions. For example, the apportioning of breast cancers into subtypes is becoming the standard of practice in clinical diagnosis. One such subtype is defined in part by the overexpression of the oncogene ERBB2 which encodes the Human Epidermal Growth Factor Receptor 2 protein (HER2). The overexpression of this gene is responsible for approximately 30% of breast cancers. Overexpression of this receptor results in especially aggressive tumors and generally poor prognosis (Tan & Yu, 2007). The gene ERBB2 is a member of a family of human epidermal growth factor receptors that when activated result in anti-apoptosis and increased cell proliferation. Given this understanding of the underlying molecular mechanisms of this specific subclass of tumors, new drugs have been developed to target and block the HER2 receptor. The monoclonal antibody trastuzumab is one of the first drugs approved by the Food and Drug Administration based upon genomic individualization of disease. With advances such as this becoming ever more commonplace, it is difficult to envision the practice of interprofessional, patient-centered, contemporary healthcare without some fundamental knowledge about genetics and genomics and their significant role in health, wellness, and disease.

Competent delivery of care will require individual healthcare professionals and teams to have a working knowledge of the human genome and pharmacogenomics in order to facilitate patient- and family-centered care with a focus on optimizing health outcomes and reducing costs. The training of healthcare professionals in genomics represents the greatest limitation to the application of modern genetic information in patient care.

If "genomics-based healthcare is to become the norm," all healthcare professionals will need to know the fundamentals of a number of relatively recent concepts—specifically, that the genome of an organism encompasses all the genetic material in the cell. In humans, this would include the 3 billion base pairs of DNA contained in 23 pairs of chromosomes in the nucleus and the approximately 16,000 base pairs of the mitochondria. Humans have approximately 23,000 functioning genes and a nearly equal number of nonfunctioning genes (pseudogenes), the remnants of past mutational events. Genomics is the study of genome structure and organization. Genomics also seeks to understand how the genome changes through time and the role of these changes in gene regulation and function. One of the most dominant areas within the field of genomics is pharmacogenetics and pharmacogenomics. Pharmacogenetics is the study of the role of human genetic variation in determining individual drug response. Generally, pharmacogenetics has been limited to the effects of one or a few genes. Pharmacogenomics, on the other hand, is the study of the genome-wide role of human variation in drug response. Pharmacogenomics is a broader term and includes pharmacogenetic effects. Pharmacogenomics also includes the application of genomic technologies in drug discovery, disposition, and function (National Human Genome Research Institute, 2014a. Frequently asked questions about pharmacogenomics: http://www.genome.gov/27530645).

While to many the fields of pharmacogenetics and pharmacogenomics seem relatively recent disciplines the term "pharmacogenetics" was actually coined in 1959 by Friedrich Vogel (1959) some 94 years after Gregor Johann Mendel first proposed a series of rules that explained the inheritance of a number of simple traits observed in garden pea plants. Even earlier than the first definition of the term, Sir Archibald Garrod (1909) had proposed in his book, *Inborn Factors in Diseases,* the link between genetics and pharmacology, postulating that a mutation in a gene could be responsible for differences among patients in enzyme metabolism. Amazingly, this was many years before DNA was tentatively identified as the molecule that carries genetic instructions in living things (NHGRI Talking Glossary http://www.genome.gov/Glossary/index. cfm?id=48; for an excellent review of the history of pharmacogenetics see Kalow, 2004). In 1962, the first book was published describing the role of human genetic variations in explaining drug response among humans (Kalow, 1962). Similar to most of modern medicine, the field of pharmacogenetics grew slowly until the advent of molecular biology and our ability to study individual genes and determine their sequence. With the completion of the Human Genome Project, the field of pharmacogenomics was born and quickly became one of the most advanced fields within the realm of "genomics."

Knowledge about the human genome and advances in pharmacogenetics and pharmacogenomics are now leading modern healthcare toward truly personalized medicine. Personalized medicine involves the application of molecular genetic tools to tailor medical treatment and therapeutics to each individual patient's needs during all stages of care (National Human Genome Research Institute, 2014b). Our growing knowledge of the human genome and the genetic differences among us is also allowing for the personalization of preventive care. While the identification of specific mutations rarely proves definitive in predicting an individual's risk of disease, with a few notable exceptions (sickle cell anemia and cystic fibrosis, for example), knowledge of the presence of some mutations allows for an assessment of risk for a patient and the possibility of taking precautions to minimize that risk. As our knowledge of the human genome grows, and with the advent of next-generation sequencing technologies, the role of genomics in guiding therapy and perhaps preventing or alleviating some of the harm for many diseases will be possible.

Who Should Read This Book

The purpose of this book is to provide readers, both nursing students and practitioners, with the foundational knowledge of the basic principles of human genetics and genomics such that they can then apply this knowledge base to challenges in optimizing drug therapy and patient care. This book provides a concise source of the basics of pharmacogenetics and pharmacogenomics such that the reader will be able to understand and make use of genetic information as the field continues to grow.

This book is geared to nursing students, educators, and practitioners with an educational goal of providing the essentials for successful practice in a healthcare environment that will be increasingly focused on the use of pharmacogenetics and pharmacogenomics in a patient-centered-practice interprofessional model.

Book Content

Given the potential differences in experience of our intended readers, from students to new practitioners to practitioners with many years of experience, the book chapters are organized as a progression through the evolving field of pharmacogenomics. Each chapter is intended to be relatively independent of the others. The first four chapters introduce the necessary basic genetic principles and concepts that underlie pharmacogenomics (Chapter 1), a brief primer on the technologies that are driving the field of pharmacogenomics (Chapter 2), the basic principles of pharmacogenetics (Chapter 3) and the implications of pharmacogenomics for the practice of nursing (Chapter 4). Chapters 5 through 9 use these basic concepts presented in the first four chapters to explore in more depth the specific areas encountered in the practice of obstetrics and prenatal care (Chapter 5), pediatrics (Chapter 6), geriatrics (Chapter 7), and oncology (Chapter 8). Chapter 9 examines the ethical considerations for nurses involved in integrating genetics and genomics into modern healthcare. Students who are familiar with the basics of genetics and genomics may move to the later chapters immediately and may refer back to the introductory chapters if necessary. Chapter 10 summarizes the need and methodologies for the introduction of pharmacogenomics in interprofessional education. Finally, Chapter 11 explores the future of medicine and healthcare in a world dominated by genomic information. Each chapter starts with a list of learning objectives that we hope the reader will be able to master upon completion of the chapter. At the end of the chapters are a series of questions to test the comprehension of the reader.

Final Thoughts

As noted earlier, the practice of medicine in the very immediate future will require of all health professionals the ability to understand and, more importantly, to accurately communicate and interpret pharmacogenomic information to the patient. The essential competencies in pharmacogenomics encompass much more than a knowledge of specific drugs and the identified genes that play a role in their metabolism or disposition, genes that code for therapeutic targets. As a member of the healthcare team, nurses must acquire the appropriate competency in pharmacogenomics in order to carry out their role of optimizing and enhancing their patient's healthcare.

Driven largely by continuing technological advances, the application of genetic or genomic principles to our understanding of human health has and will continue to revolutionize the nature of healthcare and the standards of practice for healthcare providers at all levels and professional settings. This book is designed as a reference to provide nursing students and practitioners with the essential foundational knowledge that can be used in interpreting current and future peer-reviewed publications and clinical protocols encountered in contemporary and future practice settings.

–Dale Halsey Lea, MPH, RN, GCG, APNG
dlea@maine.rr.com

–Dennis J. Cheek, PhD, RN, FAHA
d.cheek@tcu.edu

–Daniel Brazeau, PhD
dbrazeau@une.edu

–Gayle Brazeau, PhD
gbrazeau@une.edu

References

Garrod, A. E. (1909). *The inborn errors of metabolism.* London, UK: Oxford University Press.

Kalow, W. (1962). *Pharmacogenetics: Heredity and the response to drugs.* Philadelphia, London: W. B. Saunders.

Kalow, W. (2004). Pharmacogenetics: A historical perspective. In S. J. Thomas (Ed.), *Pharmacogenomics: Applications to patient care* (pp. 251–269). Kansas City, MO: American College of Clinical Pharmacy.

National Human Genome Research Institute (2014a). Frequently asked questions about pharmacogenomics. Retrieved from http://www.genome.gov/27530645

National Human Genome Research Institute (2014b). Talking glossary of genetic terms: Personalized medicine. Retrieved from http://www.genome.gov/Glossary/index.cfm?id=48

Tan, M., & Yu, D. (2007). Molecular mechanisms of erbB2-mediated breast cancer chemoresistance. *Advances in Experimental Medicine and Biology*, 608, 119–29.

Vogel, F. (1959). Probleme der Humangenetik. *Ergebnisse der inneren Medizin und Kinderheilkunde*, 12, 65–126.

Basics of Genetics and Genomics

Dale Halsey Lea, MPH, RN, CGC, APNG
Chris Winkelman, PhD, RN, CCRN, ACNP, CNE, FCCM

1

Introduction to Pharmacogenomics

Pharmacogenomics—which uses genetic data to improve prediction of a patient's responses to drugs while avoiding adverse drug reactions—supports a personalized approach to healthcare. The opportunities for adoption of pharmacogenomics testing in a variety of clinical situations are increasing (Caudle et al., 2014). Combining the science of pharmacology with the science of the human genome to choose drugs and drug doses that are effective with minimal adverse effects is helping to manage cardiovascular disease, cancer, asthma, depression, and many other common conditions (National Human Genome Research Institute, 2014g). In the current regulated market, a drug may be more likely to meet regulatory approval if the efficacy or safety in a known subpopulation identified through genomic testing benefited from the dose. Further, direct-to-consumer tests target testing of an individual's genome, and pharmacogenomic tests may be requested by patients (Patrinos, Baker, Al-Mulla, Vasiliou, & Cooper, 2013).

Put another way, pharmacogenetics is the individual inheritance of DNA (deoxyribonucleic acid) sequences that contributes to individual response to drugs. In 2008, the United States Food and Drug Administration (FDA), which is the agency responsible for national drug approval, defined pharmacogenetics as

OBJECTIVES

- Pharmacogenomics is creating a personalized approach to healthcare.

- Combining the sciences of pharmacology with the human genome to choose effective drugs and drug doses is helping to manage many acute and chronic conditions.

- A person's genetic material provides clinicians with essential information to evaluate individual variation in drug response.

- Nurses need to be knowledgeable about the role of genetic materials, such as deoxyriboncleic acid (DNA), ribonucleic acid (RNA), genes, and gene expression in drug metabolism.

the study of variations in DNA sequence as related to drug response (U.S. FDA, 2008, p. 3). Pharmacogenomics, according to the same document, is the study of variations of DNA and RNA (ribonucleic acid) characteristics as related to drug response, implying that protein products resulting from gene activity contribute to individual drug response. Currently, terminology favors the use of the pharmacogenomics to describe hereditary influences of variation between individuals in response to a specific drug (Ventola, 2011a).

Substantial variability occurs when individuals are given the same drug. Patients who respond positively to a drug range from 30% to 60% (Bhathena & Spear, 2008; Kisor, Kane, Talbot, & Sprague, 2014). Effective response to drugs for cancer treatment can be as low as 25% (Gillis, Patel, & Innocenti, 2014). Additionally, individuals experience idiosyncratic and unpredictable toxic and adverse effects from drugs. Multiple factors contribute to variable drug responses including adherence, age, body mass index (BMI), presence and severity of comorbidities/illnesses, drug-drug and drug-food interactions, and the surrounding environment. Genetic research since the mapping of the human genome in 2003 has generated extensive knowledge about how DNA, RNA, proteins, and metabolites affect drug responses (Ventola, 2011a). Genomics is estimated to contribute to 20% to 50% of an individual's drug response; the range varies between drugs and drug classes.

Ventola (2011b) cited growing demands to personalize medicine, including the use of pharmacogenomic testing, reflected in direct-to-consumer advertising. The clinician who administers and prescribes drugs needs to build understanding about the utility, feasibility, and ethical and societal implications of pharmacogenomic testing for individualizing drug therapy.

The implications of pharmacogenomics for clinical nursing practice are addressed in each chapter. This chapter provides an overview of genetics and genomics related to pharmacology. Throughout the text, concepts are linked to examples from pharmacogenomic findings. Content in this chapter includes a review of the genetic and genomic information, including the structure and function of genes and an explanation of genetic diversity that forms the basis of pharmacogenomic testing and application of results as illustrated in the scenario that follows.

PHARMACOGENOMICS IN ACTION

May is a 72-year-old woman with hypertension, hyperlipidemia, and severe peripheral arterial disease (PAD) of both legs who lives with minimal assistance in an older adult urban residence. Last week, she was admitted to the emergency department (ED) with new onset dyspnea and profound fatigue. Diagnostic studies confirmed an evolving myocardial infarction. She was urgently transported to the facility's cardiac catheterization lab. A 90% left anterior descending coronary artery occlusion was managed with the insertion of a single intracoronary artery stent. After an uncomplicated inpatient stay, she was discharged with most of her prehospitalization prescriptions continued. However, clopidogrel, her previously prescribed antiplatelet drug, was stopped; and a new agent, prasugrel (Effient) was prescribed. When May went to fill this new prescription at her community pharmacy, she learned that the new drug cost $81 for a 30-day supply compared with $10 for clopidogrel. She did not fill the prescription and called you, her primary care nurse practitioner (NP), to ask that clopidogrel be continued. She has a one-week supply of the new drug and will take it while you investigate patient-centered options.

You call the cardiologist who performed the angiography and stent placement, expecting the provider to agree to the change, given that clopidogrel is often prescribed following stent placement in your other patients. However, the cardiologist states that it is unlikely that clopidogrel will work well in this particular patient because she developed an intracoronary artery thrombosis while receiving clopidogrel. As many as 20% of patients do not receive a benefit from clopidogrel.

You immediately schedule a pharmacogenomic test to determine May's genetic profile and address concerns about selection of an effective drug. The pharmacogenomic test is paid for through May's insurer, Medicare (http://cms.hhs.gov), and includes the analysis of nine common cytochrome P450 (CYP) enzymes involved in drug metabolism. The pharmacogenomic test reveals that May is a slow CYP2C19 metabolizer. This result confirms the cardiologist's clinical decision: namely, that clopidogrel—a prodrug—is unlikely to be effective in the prevention of thromboses for May. A prodrug is a medication that needs to be converted to an active form. Typically, conversion occurs through metabolism in the liver. Slow metabolizers do not convert sufficient quantities of clopidogrel to an active antiplatelet agent; slow metabolizers of clopidogrel are at increased risk for cardiovascular events after stent placement (Price, 2012). Prasugrel is an active drug that is deactivated by CYP3A4 and 2B6 enzymes, with minor involvement of the 2C19 enzymes (U.S. FDA, 2014a). Because there is essentially no genetic variability associated with CYP3A4 enzymes, and because the results of May's pharmacogenomic test reveal no concerns about 2B6, you note that prasugrel is likely to be effective at the usual dose and without increased toxicity risk for this individual.

Because May's concerns are about affordability, you next contact the manufacturer of prasugrel and successfully enroll her in a program to decrease her out-of-pocket costs. She registers for cardiac rehabilitation, recovers uneventfully from her acute coronary event, and experiences no complications from severe PAD while on her revised antiplatelet regimen. As the primary care NP, your knowledge of pharmacology and pharmacogenomics has ensured that May's care is congruent with patient-centered outcomes and reflects current practice recommendations.

Genetic Materials in Humans That Influence Individual Variation in Drug Responses

Understanding how our genetic material works provides the clinician with essential information about individual variation in drug response. It is important for nurses to be knowledgeable about the role of genetic materials, such as deoxyribonucleic acid (DNA), ribonucleic acid (RNA), genes, and gene expression in drug metabolism. Transcription and translation of proteins generated by genes also influence the individual's response to drugs.

Deoxyribonucleic Acid

Deoxyribonucleic acid (DNA) is the hereditary material in humans and almost all other organisms (Genetics Home Reference, 2014f). The majority of human DNA is found in the cell nucleus. Additional DNA in the cell mitochondria provides instructions for the energy functions of the mitochondria (i.e., oxidative phosphorylation) as well as the codes for making molecules of RNA essential to assembling amino acids into functional proteins.

DNA is made of four base pairs with alternating sugar and phosphate groups: adenine, cytosine, guanine, and thymine. DNA stores the information for protein synthesis. An alteration in a DNA base may lead to a change in protein structure or the stability of the protein, or impact protein activity and alter the function of drugs or host response. Proteins involved in pharmacokinetics include transporters in the gastrointestinal and other systems (absorption); carriers in the bloodstream (distribution); enzymes in drug degradation (metabolism); and transporters in the tubules of the kidney (elimination). Proteins that move drugs across cell membranes, act as solute carriers, activate prodrugs and metabolize (deactivate) active drugs, and contribute to drug excretion are all manufactured in cells, using a template provided by DNA.

DNA also codes for proteins essential to pharmacodynamics, including cell membrane receptors, such as beta adrenergic receptors that bind norepinephrine, and enzymes, such as 5-lipoxygenase, that promote leukotriene formation. Individuals with DNA sequences that result in reduced synthesis of beta-adrenergic receptors are less responsive to albuterol (AccuNab, ProAir, Proventil, Ventolin, generic), which is an inhaled drug used to manage bronchoconstriction during asthma exacerbation and other lung conditions. Individuals with low 5-lipoxygenase production do not experience the same effective prevention of bronchoconstriction from drugs such as zileutin (Zyflo; a drug that blocks 5-lipoxygenase production) compared with individuals with "wild type" genes producing normal or common levels of 5-lipoxygenase.

Ribonucleic Acid

Ribonucleic acid (RNA) is a single-stranded molecule with a structure of alternating sugar (ribose) and phosphate groups similar to DNA with the substitution of uracil for thymine for one base (National Human Genome Research Institute, 2014g). RNA transfers the code for protein building from the cell's nucleus to the ribosomes where proteins are synthesized. Three types of RNA participate in the protein-synthesizing pathway in all cells. In addition, there is noncoding RNA involved in regulating whether a gene is "turned on" to generate a protein or "turned off."

The three types of RNA essential to protein synthesis are

- **Messenger RNA (mRNA):** The mRNA leaves the cell nucleus with a transcription of the genetic code for a protein and moves to the cytoplasm, where proteins are made.
- **Ribosomal RNA (rRNA):** During protein synthesis, the ribosome moves along the mRNA, reads its base sequence, and uses the genetic code to translate each three-base triplet, or *codon*, into its corresponding amino acid (National Human Genome Research Institute, 2014j). Ribosomal RNA makes up the large and small subunits of a ribosome, "reading" the base sequence of the mRNA

and interacting with the tRNAs to build the protein derived from the DNA code.

- **Transfer RNA (tRNA):** Transfer RNA contributes to protein synthesis through the formation of a complementary sequence to the mRNA molecule, ensuring that the appropriate amino acid is inserted into the protein (Genetics Home Reference, 2014c).

DNA has four chemicals that form its basic structure, or bases: adenine (A), guanine (G), cytosine (C), and thymine (T). Similarly, RNA has four chemical bases. Three bases are the same as found in DNA; the exception is uracil (U) in place of thymine. The sequence of these bases directs the formation of protein. DNA and RNA contain other chemicals, such as phosphate groups, proteins, and sugars, which contribute to the shape and function of DNA and RNA.

In DNA and RNA, a sequence of three bases—or nucleotides—will code for a certain amino acid. The series of three bases coding for one amino acid is known as a *codon*. Ultimately, codons combine to provide a genetic code that is a recipe for a protein sequence. There are 64 different codons, of which 61 specify amino acids and three are used as stop signals. Combinations of the codons provide all the information to build the proteins that, in turn, construct cell components, cells, tissues, organs, systems, and human beings. (Genetics Home Reference, 2014a).

Genes

A *gene* is a segment of DNA that codes for a specific protein. Genes vary in size from a few hundred DNA bases to more than 2 million bases. Findings from the Human Genome Project resulted in an estimated 20,000 to 25,000 genes present in humans (Genetics Home Reference, 2014g). A *genome* is the entire set of genetic instructions found in a cell. In humans, the genome consists of 23 pairs of chromosomes, found in the nucleus, as well as the genes in mitochondria.

A "wild type" gene is the most common or prevalent sequence of DNA in a population (Korf & Irons, 2013). Variations in the sequence of wild type genes can lead to a change in protein structure or stability. This change in protein, in turn, can lead to an unanticipated or alternate patient response to drugs.

Genes may account for 20% or more of drug effects as well as how drugs are handled by the body (Korf & Irons, 2013). The genes that code for the cytochrome P450 (CYP450) enzymes are examples of DNA sequences that have important effects on drug metabolism. The CYP450 enzymes are able to break down more than half of drugs used to manage diseases and conditions, including warfarin, a drug that is used to prevent blood clots. CYP450 enzymes also activate prodrugs, or compounds that must undergo metabolism before exerting effects on the human body. Variations in the CYP450 genes can influence how well an individual's body is able to metabolize certain drugs or activate prodrugs. For example, a single dose of a particular drug can have a profound effect in those individuals who have a less active form of the enzyme, contributing to toxic effects from prolonged circulation of the drug, as if receiving excess dosing over time. Alternatively, individuals who have a more active form of the enzyme may appear to have a low or lack of response due to rapid breakdown of the drug, resulting in a need for more frequent dosing or a larger dose to obtain a therapeutic response (National Human Genome Research Institute, 2014c).

Another example of metabolic proteins related to pharmacology is the gene that codes for uridine diphosphate glucuronosyltransferase (UGT1A1), which is an enzyme produced in the liver that deactivates irinotecan (Camptpsar), a drug used for palliative management of colorectal cancer (Paulik, Grim, & Filip, 2012). Treatment with irinotecan can cause severe neutropenia and diarrhea. The majority of these adverse drug reactions are caused by the insufficient deactivation (glucuronidation) of irinotecan (Paulik et al., 2012). Since 2005, the FDA has recommended pharmacogenomic testing of individuals in advance of administering the drug to avoid life-threatening toxicities (Paulik et al., 2012).

Additional exemplars are related to drug transporters (distribution) and drug excretory channels (elimination). One potential explanation for individuals with chronic seizure disorder who do not respond to anti-epileptic drugs is the excess production of P-glycoprotein, which is a membrane transporter produced in secretory cells of the liver, small intestine, renal tubules, and endothelium of brain capillaries (Stepien, Tomaszewski, Tomaszewska, & Czuczwar, 2012). P-glycoprotein acts as a drug efflux pump, reducing the transfer of drugs into cells; it is thought to prevent the accumulation of anti-epileptic drugs in brain cells (Stepien et al., 2012). The last example of genetic coding that affects drug response occurs in renal tubules. Organic ion transporters contribute to the elimination of many drugs, including metformin, a drug commonly used to manage Type 2 diabetes. Some inherited differences in the code for construction and activity of ion transporters are thought to contribute to reduced effectiveness and increased toxicity following metformin administration (Zolk, 2012). Patients with a specific *cation* (positive ion) transporter are more likely to experience lactic acidosis with concurrent use of metformin during renal insufficiency.

Gene Expression, Transcription, and Translation

Even when genes have the correct code, errors can be made in protein formation that contribute to adverse drug effects. Genes can also be silenced ("turned off"), causing reductions in protein formation, or induced ("turned on") to create abnormally high volumes of harmful proteins. Gene silencing is a subspecialty of *epigenetics* (genetic investigation). These processes of genetic activity are also the focus of pharmacogenetic and pharmacogenomic investigation and targets for drug development.

Gene expression is the process by which the information encoded in a gene is used to direct the assembly of a protein molecule. The cell reads the sequence of the gene in groups of three bases. Each group of three bases (codon) corresponds to one of 20 different amino acids used to build a protein (National Human Genome Research Institute, 2014d). Instructions stored in the DNA are expressed in two steps: transcription and translation.

Gene transcription is the step that converts DNA to RNA (Genetics Home Reference, 2014b). RNA may be the final product when the RNA is used for an intracellular function. Few errors typically occur during transcription. More often, the RNA formed in the nucleus serves a template for mRNA and instructions for the next step, translation. One target for drug development is to induce transcription when a deficit of protein is causing a disease, such as the malformed chloride transporter for patients with cystic fibrosis.

Translation is the process by which the base sequence of an mRNA is used to organize and join amino acids into a protein; it is the conversion of mRNA into protein (Genetics Home Reference, 2014d). Translation occurs in a process of initiation, elongation, and termination in ribosomes. Although errors are not common during this process, they do occur. One type of error is a "stop" error, whereby the mRNA has a codon that signals for the premature cessation of protein formation, resulting in a truncated protein that is ineffective or harmful. Nonstop errors can lead to folding or formation errors such that the protein has reduced or nonexistent activity in the case of a drug-metabolizing enzyme. Nonstop errors can also cause ribosomes to lose the ability to release factors needed to allow the protein to leave the ribosome, such as the case of a fully formed drug receptor protein not leaving the ribosome to be incorporated into a cell membrane, decreasing the potential for drug-receptor interaction and drug effectiveness.

Some drugs target gene expression. One example is imatinib (Gleevec), which is a drug used to manage chronic myeloid leukemia and acute lymphocytic leukemia caused by the abnormal Philadelphia chromosome (National Cancer Institute, 2014a). The Philadelphia chromosome produces a growth factor in bone marrow cells leading to malignancy. Imatinib inhibits the activity of tyrosine kinase, an essential enzyme for cell growth. With imatinib, myeloid cell proliferation is reduced, and apoptosis of malignant leukemic cells occurs (National Cancer Institute, 2014b).

Some drugs affect proteins after formation; the drug target is a post-translational treatment. An example of this type of drug therapy is ivacaftor (Kaylydeco; U.S. FDA, 2014b). Although ivacaftor does not directly affect transcription or translation, it does alter the folding of a defective protein coded by DNA. In people with specific genetic mutations (e.g., the G551D mutation of the CFTR gene) causing cystic fibrosis, ivacaftor improves the function of the chloride ion channel, allowing for the flow of salt and fluids across lung cells. Improved chloride ion channel structure helps to thin the thick, sticky mucus in lungs common to cystic fibrosis. More than 400 mutations of the gene that codes for chloride ion channels result in a diagnosis of cystic fibrosis (National Human Genome Research Institute, 2014k). In terms of pharmacogenomics, patients need to be tested for the specific genetic mutations that respond to invacaftor before it is prescribed and used.

Genes in Pedigrees

An individual's *pedigree* is a genetic representation of his or her family tree that illustrates the inheritance of a disease or trait through several generations. A pedigree also shows the relationships among the individual's family members and identifies which family members express or carry the trait or disease gene (National Human Genome Research Institute, 2014l). Family history, displayed in a pedigree, is an essential component of health assessment.

Mendelian Transmission Patterns

Genes are passed on from parents to their children. They contain information that is needed to specify a trait (National Human Genome Research Institute, 2014e). Some genes that children inherit from their parents may cause genetic disorders. Some of these genetic disorders may be caused by a mutation in one gene. Genes that can cause a genetic disorder can be inherited from a person's parents several ways. The basic patterns of inheritance of single gene diseases are referred to as Mendelian inheritance because Gregor Mendel identified the different patterns of gene segregation and was able to determine what the probabilities were of recurrence of a particular trait for future generations. Single genes, for example, are usually inherited in one of several patterns, which depend on the location of the gene and whether one or two copies of the gene are necessary for the disease to develop. It is now known that there are five basic modes of inheritance for single gene diseases. These are autosomal dominant, autosomal recessive, X-linked dominant, X-linked recessive, and mitochondrial (Genetic Alliance, 2008).

Autosomal Dominant Inheritance

One way a gene can cause a genetic disorder is by autosomal dominant inheritance. *Autosomal* means that the particular gene is located on one of the numbered, non-sex chromosomes. *Dominant* in this context indicates that a single copy of the gene mutation associated with the disease is sufficient to cause the particular disease (National Human Genome Research Institute, 2014b). An affected individual usually has one affected parent. Huntington's disease is an example of a disease caused by an autosomal dominant gene mutation. In pharmacogenomics, a variation in vitamin K epoxide reductase affects the production of vitamin K and, ultimately, contributes to resistance to the effectiveness of warfarin (Coumadin) when administered at a typical dose in patients who use this drug for anticoagulation (Aquilante et al., 2006). The inherited resistance can be overcome with high doses of warfarin.

Another example of autosomal inheritance helps to explain adverse severe cutaneous reactions to some drugs. The HLA-B gene (human leukocyte antigen B or major histocompatibility complex, class I, B) has hundreds of variations in humans. A few variations are associated with potentially serious and life-threatening skin reactions, ranging from Stevens-Johnson syndrome to toxic epidermal necrolysis. Skin hypersensitivity reactions can be avoided with genetic testing before starting abacivir or nevirapine (both used to treat patients with human immunodeficiency virus [HIV]) and carbamazepine (an anti-epileptic drug; Phillips, Chung, Mockenhaupt, Roujeau, & Mallal, 2011). Recall that in autosomal inheritance, a single gene conveys the susceptibility to severe cutaneous hypersensitivity reactions for these drugs.

Autosomal Recessive Inheritance

Autosomal recessive inheritance is another way genes can cause a genetic disorder. In autosomal recessive inherited disorders, two copies of a mutated gene are present in each cell. An individual who has an autosomal recessive disorder usually has parents who are unaffected but who each carry a single copy of the mutated gene. The parents are called *carriers*. Autosomal recessive genetic disorders are not usually seen in each generation of an affected family member. Cystic fibrosis is an example of an autosomal recessive genetic disorder. Patients who are categorized as "fast" or "slow" acetylators inherit this metabolic variation in an autosomal recessive manner. The N-acetyltransferase enzyme is a phase-2 liver metabolizing enzyme necessary to the breakdown of isoniazid (used to manage tuberculosis), sulfonamides (used as anti-infectives), procainamide (an antidysrhythmic), and hydralazine (an antihypertensive drug; Correia, 2012). Recall that two genes, one from each parent, need to be present to manifest cystic fibrosis or fast and slow acetylation of drugs.

X-linked Dominant Genetic Disorders

X-linked dominant genetic disorders are caused by gene mutations that are located on an X chromosome. Females are more often affected than males. The possibility of passing an X-linked dominant gene is different for males and females. A family with an X-linked dominant genetic disorder may have affected males and females in each generation. Also, fathers are not able to pass X-linked traits to their sons. Fragile X syndrome is an example of an X-linked dominant gene.

X-linked Recessive Genetic Disorders

X-linked recessive genetic disorders are also caused by gene mutations on an X chromosome. The chance to pass on the X-linked disorder is different between males and females. In those families that have an X-linked recessive disorder, males are often more affected than females (infrequently affected) in each generation. In X-linked recessive inheritance, a father does not pass the X-linked gene to his sons, so no male-to-male transmission occurs. Hemophilia is an example of an X-linked recessive genetic disorder.

Mitochondrial Inheritance

Another type of inheritance is *mitochondrial inheritance*, which is a type of maternal inheritance and involves genes in mitochondrial DNA. *Mitochondria* are structures present in each cell that are able to change molecules into energy, and each one contains a small amount of DNA. Because only a woman's egg cells can contribute mitochondria to an embryo, only females are able to pass mitochondrial gene mutations to their children. Mitochondrial disorders can be seen in each generation of a family, and both males and females can be affected. However, a father does not pass mitochondrial disorders to his children. Leber hereditary optic neuropathy is an example of a mitochondrial disorder (Genetics Home Reference, 2014e). Some drugs may affect mitochondrial function, perhaps through epigenetics or posttranslational effects. One example is propofol, an anesthetic and sedative drug (Savard, Dupré, & Brunet, 2013). Administration of propofol may protect myocardial cells from ischemic injury during cardiac surgery by interrupting the formation of free radical oxygen species (Shao et al., 2008). Free radical oxygen species are toxic to cells and cell components like mitochondria.

> **NOTE**
>
> *Quantitative genetics* is the study of the genetics of complex traits, such as obesity and size, as well as how traits vary significantly among individuals. Complex traits have continuously distributed phenotypes that do not appear to show the simple Mendelian inheritance patterns. The study of genetics and complex traits is based on a model in which a number of genes may have an influence on the trait, and in which nongenetic factors may also have an important role (Hill, 2010).

Multifactorial Inheritance

Multifactorial inheritance—a pattern of inheritance that is seen in common health conditions such as diabetes and heart disease—is caused by a combination of genes and other factors such as lifestyle, aging, and environmental factors. The inherited gene abnormalities cause an individual to be at increased risk for or susceptible to developing the condition. However, that individual may not develop the disorder unless other lifestyle and environmental factors are present. Examining an individual's family health history can help to determine whether that individual and other family members are at risk for a particular multifactorial condition. If an individual has one or more relatives with a particular health condition, and that person develops the condition at a younger age than expected, other family members may have an increased risk to develop the condition or pass it to their children (Center for Genetics Education, 2014).

The variations in pharmacodynamics and pharmacokinetics in individuals is multifactorial. Although genetic testing can provide additional, important information, it is not the only source of information the clinician will use to determine clinical efficacy and risk for adverse events from a drug. Nonetheless, the Clinical Pharmacogenetics Implementation Consortium (CPIC) has developed dosing guidelines based on pharmacogenomics in multiple drugs (Pharmacogenomics Knowledge Implementation, 2014). The CPIC provides freely available, peer-reviewed, updatable, and detailed gene-drug clinical practice guidelines.

Genomes: Diversity, Size, and Structure

An individual's *genome* is the complete set of genetic instructions located in a cell. A human's genome has 23 pairs of chromosomes, which are located in the cell nucleus. Also, a small chromosome is located in the cell's mitochondria. When taken together, all these chromosomes have approximately 3.1 billion bases of DNA sequence (National Human Genome Research Institute, 2014h).

Genetic variation, which is the differences in the genetic sequence among individuals and societies, can help to explain some of the physiological differences between individuals that may cause an increased or decreased risk for disease. Some of these diseases are caused by a single genetic difference. Common diseases, on the other hand, are usually caused by complex interactions among multiple genes as well as environmental factors (National Human Genome Research Institute, 2014j).

A number of genetic variations can occur. One type is a *mutation*, which is a change at the level of DNA when one or more base pairs have undergone a change from normal. Mutations include deletions, insertions, and genetic rearrangements that can affect several genes or large areas of a chromosome at once. Variations in DNA sequence that cause disease are often categorized as mutations, although not all mutations cause disease.

Another type of genetic variation is *polymorphism,* which also involves differences in individual DNA. Polymorphic DNA variations result in sequences that are considered equally standard or normal in populations. Generally, to be classified a polymorphism, the least common variation (also called "allele") must occur with a frequency of 1% or more in the population, and mutations occur at <1%. The most common type of polymorphism is the single nucleotide polymorphism (SNP). Another polymorphic variation is copy number variations, in which some DNA repeats itself. There can be variation in the number of repeats (National Human Genome Research Institute, 2014f).

Polymorphic variations usually do not cause obvious disease. However, this type of DNA variation can contribute to disease susceptibility and influences drug response. For example, a deficiency of an enzyme needed to break down a chemical that gives fish an unpleasant odor is also used to breakdown nicotine. Several different variations in the enzyme's gene sequence result in either loss of the enzyme or reduced function, causing a body malodor when fish or lecithin-rich substances are consumed (Yamazaki & Shimizu, 2007). Although malodor is an unpleasant condition (rather than a disease), this inherited condition could be classed as a mutation when malodor is extreme, or a polymorphism if the condition is mild and avoidable with dietary adjustments. The variations (causing absent or reduced enzyme synthesis) would also slow the metabolism of nicotine, resulting in a possible aversion to tobacco from sustained gastrointestinal effects (e.g., nausea, hypermotility), so it may even be considered a "protective" genetic variant!

> **NOTE**
>
> The rules around categorization of a genetic variation are neither hard nor fast, with great overlaps classifying a DNA sequence variation as a mutation or polymorphism (National Human Genome Research Institute, 2014a).

Structural genomic variants (SGVs) range in size from the large and microscopically visible chromosome aberrations to variants of the DNA sequence level, such as small insertions or deletions of several base pairs. SGVs are found among all humans and are likely to contribute significantly to an individual's susceptibility to diseases. The most common form of SGV is *copy number variants* (CNVs), which are defined as segments that are greater than 1 kilobase (kb) in length and that exist in variable copy numbers between individuals (Smith et al., 2008)

Genetic Mapping: Genome-Wide Association Studies

As a result of the completion of the Human Genome Project in 2003 and the International HapMap Project in 2005, research tools are available that make it possible to identify the genetic contributions to common diseases. The tools include a map of human genetic variation and new technologies that can accurately and rapidly analyze whole genome samples to identify genetic variations that can contribute to the development of a particular disease. Genome-wide association studies (GWAS) are one of these studies that are now possible. GWAS uses rapidly scanning markers throughout complete genomes of many individuals to identify genetic variations that are associated with a type of disease. Researchers can then use this information to create better ways to identify, treat, and prevent a particular disease. These GWAS are becoming very useful in identifying genetic variations that can cause common and complex disorders such as heart disease, diabetes, cancer, and asthma.

Genome-wide association studies are expected to have a significant influence on medical care by creating the groundwork for a new type of medicine called "personalized medicine." As improvements are made on the efficiency and the cost of GWAS, healthcare professionals will be able to use these tools to individualize patients' information about their risks to develop a particular disease. And GWAS will make it possible for healthcare professionals to create disease preventions that are based on their patient's specific genetic makeup. If the patient develops the particular disorder, his or her genetic makeup can be used to choose the treatments that will be most effective (National Human Genome Research Institute, 2014i).

> For more on genome-wide association studies, visit:
> www.genome.gov/gwastudies

Implementation of Genetic Testing in Personalized Medicine

The identification of DNA sequence variations that are associated with individual drug response is increasing. Although clinical pharmacogenetic testing is not yet widely used, it is available in both Clinical Laboratory Improvement Amendment (CLIA)–certified laboratories and other settings. Genetic tests are directly available to consumers (direct-to-consumer genetic tests). Direct-to-consumer genetic tests are advertised on consumer medical education sites and may or may not have a component of counseling or expert interpretation of results packaged with the test fee. When the burden of drug therapy is high, such as with the toxicity of drugs used to manage HIV or provide HIV prophylaxis, consumers may turn to direct-to-consumer genetic tests to screen for the potential of adverse drug effects (like HLA-B variations) or to evaluate the efficacy of a drug.

The advances in genetic testing technology like GWAS and the rapid turnaround in results are enhancing clinical application of genetic testing for personalized use of drugs (Abdul-Husn, Obeng, Sanderson, Gottesman, & Scott, 2014). Clinical practice guidelines for pharmacogenetic results are currently available in selected drugs. Direct-to-consumer pharmacogenetic testing will also contribute to consumer awareness of genetic variations that result in drug response or adverse drug events and impact nursing practice. Nurses and advanced practice nurses must be able to apply information about genetics and pharmacogenetic testing to provide safe, effective options for therapeutic drugs (as with drugs used to manage cancer).

Summary

People experience a wide range of response to drugs. Knowledge of a patient's genome is used to evaluate drug efficacy and avoid toxicity in a variety of clinical conditions, and it is increasingly providing an explanation for variable drug response. Pharmacogenomics references the science and methods that investigate all genes involved in the response to a drug. Pharmacogenomic testing uses individual genomic biomarkers to choose the ideal drug and/or dose for a patient, with the goal of optimizing efficacy while avoiding toxicity and adverse drug reactions.

Understanding how an individual's genome results in a variable response to a drug or dose has limited but important clinical applicability today, but the application of genomic and genetic information to personalize drug selection is expected to become increasingly common and useful to clinical practice. Pharmacogenomics is contributing to drug discovery and targeted drug use by using GWAS to identify biomarkers that recognize individuals most likely to respond and those at greatest risk for harm from prescribed drugs.

All healthcare professionals should know about the interaction of genetic factors that influences response to treatment (NCHPEG, 2007). Knowledge of pharmacogenetics and pharmacogenomics is a core competency essential to all healthcare professionals and an essential component of basic and advanced nursing education and practice (Consensus Panel, 2008).

Questions

When does a pedigree alert the clinician to a concerning genetic pattern?

a. Whenever there is only one generation with any multifactorial condition

b. Whenever there are two generations with potentially inheritable conditions

c. Whenever there are two or more first-degree relatives sharing an inheritable condition. *

d. Whenever there is a problem with cytochrome P450 metabolism of drugs

For which of the following patients is there significant evidence that genetic testing related to metabolizing enzymes provides benefit?

a. The patient with tuberculosis receiving rifampine

b. The patient with coronary artery disease receiving clopidogrel *

c. The patient with cancer receiving imatinib

d. Any patient receiving prescribed medications

Describe the feasibility and utility of using genetic testing today to provide safe, effective doses.

Tests used to measure common metabolic enzymes and the VKOPRC1 pathway are currently feasible and reimbursable by Medicare and most third party insurers. There are nine approved indications for genetic testing related to prescribed drugs. Results from these tests can avoid complications from some antidepressants, antiplatelet drugs, and warfarin, used for anticoagulation.

Key Points

- Pharmacogenomics is the study of variations of DNA and RNA characteristics as they relate to drug responses.
- Pharmacogenomic testing is the analysis of an individual's genome, or entire set of genes, with the goal of identifying variations (polymorphisms) that contribute to that individual's response to drugs.
- Pharmacogenetics is the study of how an individual's actions and reactions to drugs vary as a result of the person's genes.
- Genetic variation contributes to both pharmacokinetics and pharmacodynamics.
  - Pharmacokinetics is the process of drug absorption, distribution, metabolism, and elimination.
  - Pharmacodynamics is the interaction between drugs and drug receptors or other cellular targets.
- Traits such as resistance to drug effects or susceptibility to drug toxicity can be inherited.
  - Inherited patterns in the health history, often drawn by a pedigree, can be Mendelian or multifactorial.
  - Mendelian traits are inherited in autosomal dominant or autosomal recessive, or linked to the X-chromosome.
  - Multifactorial inheritance is the result of genes and other factors such as lifestyle, aging, and the environment.
- As findings from genome-wide association studies accumulate, pharmacogenomics is expected to become increasingly useful in identifying variations in genes that decrease drug effects or cause severe adverse drug effects.

References

Abdul-Husn, N. S., Obeng, A. O., Sanderson, S. C., Gottesman, O., Scott, S. A. (2014). Implementation and utilization of genetic testing in personalized medicine. *Pharamocgenomics and Personalized Medicine, 7*(open access), 227–240.

Aquilante, C., Langaee, T., Lopez, L., Yarandi, H., Tromberg, J., Mohuczy, D., . . . Johnson, J. (2006). Pharmacogenetics and genomics: Influence of coagulation factor, vitamin K epoxide reductase complex subunit 1, and cytochrome P450 2C9 gene polymorphisms on warfarin dose requirements. *Clinical Pharmacology & Therapeutics, 79*, 291–302.

Bhathena, A., & Spear, B. B. (2008). Pharmacogenetics: improving drug and dose selection. *Current Opinion in Pharmacology, 8*(5), 639–646. doi: 10.1016/j.coph.2008.07.013

Caudle, K. E., Klein, T. E., Hoffman, J. M., Muller, D. J., Whirl-Carrillo, M., Gong, L., . . . Johnson, S. G. (2014). Incorporation of pharmacogenomics into routine clinical practice: the Clinical Pharmacogenetics Implementation Consortium (CPIC) guideline development process. *Current Drug Metabolism, 15*(2), 209–217. Retrieved from http://www.ncbi.nlm.nih.gov/pubmed/24479687

Center for Genetics Education. (2014). Fact Sheet 11: Environmental and genetic interactions—complex patterns of inheritance 1. Retrieved from http://www.genetics.edu.au/Publications-and-Resources/Genetics-Fact-Sheets

Consensus Panel. (2008). *Essentials of Genetic and Genomic Nursing: Competencies, curricula Guidelines, and Outcome Indicators* J. J. & K. Calzone (Eds.), (pp. 80). Retrieved from http://www.nursingworld.org/MainMenuCategories/EthicsStandards/Genetics-1/EssentialNursingCompetenciesandCurriculaGuidelinesforGeneticsandGenomics.pdf

Correia, M. A. (2012). Drug Biotransformation: Introduction. In M. A. Katzung (Ed.), *Basic and Clinical Pharmacology* (12th ed.). St. Louis, MO: Appleton Lange.

Genetic Alliance. (2008). Understanding Genetics: A District of Columbia Guide for Patients and Health Professionals. Retrieved from http://www.ncbi.nlm.nih.gov/books/NBK132145/

Genetics Home Reference. (2014a). Codon. *Handbook.* Retrieved from http://ghr.nlm.nih.gov/glossary=codon

Genetics Home Reference. (2014b). Transcription. *Handbook.* Retrieved from http://ghr.nlm.nih.gov/glossary=transcription

Genetics Home Reference. (2014c). Transfer RNA. *Handbook.* Retrieved from http://www.genome.gov/glossary/index.cfm?id=123

Genetics Home Reference. (2014d). Translation. *Handbook.* Retrieved from http://ghr.nlm.nih.gov/glossary=translation

Genetics Home Reference. (2014e). What are the different ways in which a genetic conditon can be inheritied? *Handbook.* Retrieved from http://ghr.nlm.nih.gov/handbook/inheritance/inheritancepatterns

Genetics Home Reference. (2014f). What is DNA? *Handbook.* Retrieved from http://ghr.nlm.nih.gov/handbook/basics/dna

Genetics Home Reference. (2014g) What is a gene? *Handbook.* Retrieved from http://ghr.nlm.nih.gov/handbook/basics/gene

Gillis, N. K., Patel, J. N., & Innocenti, F. (2014). Clinical implementation of germ line cancer pharmacogenetic variants during the next-generation sequencing era. *Clinical Pharmacology and Therapeutics, 95*(3), 269–280. doi: 10.1038/clpt.2013.214

Hill, W. G. (2010). Understanding and using quantitative genetic variation. *Philosophical Transactions of the Royal Society of London Biological Sciences, 365*(1537), 73–85. doi: 10.1098/rstb.2009.0203

Kisor, D. F., Kane, M. D., Talbot, J. N., & Sprague, J. E. (2014). *Pharmacogenetics, kinetics, and dynamics for personalized medicine*. Burlington, MA: Jones & Bartlett.

Korf, B. R., & Irons, M. B. (2013). *Human genetics and genomics* (4th ed.). Hoboken, NJ: Wiley-Blackwell.

National Cancer Institute. (2014a). *NCI Dictionary of Cancer Terms*. Philadelphia Chromosome. Retrieved from http://www.cancer.gov/dictionary?cdrid=44179

National Cancer Institute. (2014b). *NCI Drug Dictionary*. imatinib mesylate. Retrieved from http://www.cancer.gov/drugdictionary?CdrID=37862

National Coalition for Health Professional Education in Genetics (NCHPEG). (2007). *Core competencies in genetics essential for all health-care professionals* (3rd ed.). Lutherville, MD: Author.

National Human Genome Research Institute (2014a). All about the Human Genome Project. Retrieved from http://www.genome.gov/10001772

National Human Genome Research Institute. (2014b). Autosomal dominant. *Talking Glossary of Genetic Terms*. Retrieved from https://www.genome.gov/Glossary/index.cfm?id=12

National Human Genome Research Institute. (2014c). *Frequently asked questions about genetic testing*. Retrieved from http://www.genome.gov/19516567

National Human Genome Research Institute. (2014d). Gene Expression. *Talking Glossary of Genetic Terms*. Retrieved from http://www.genome.gov/Glossary/index.cfm?id=73

National Human Genome Research Institute. (2014e). Genes. *Talking Glossary of Genetic Terms*. Retrieved from http://www.genome.gov/Glossary/index.cfm?id=70

National Human Genome Research Institute. (2014f). *Genetic Variation*. Retrieved from http://www.genome.gov/Pages/Education/Modules/GeneticVariation.pdf

National Human Genome Research Institute. (2014g). Genetics and Genomics for Patients and the Public. Frequently Asked Questions about Pharmacogenomics. Retrieved from http://www.genome.gov/27530645

National Human Genome Research Institute. (2014h). Genome. *Talking Glossary of Genetic Terms*. Retrieved from http://www.genome.gov/Glossary/index.cfm?id=90

National Human Genome Research Institute. (2014i). *Genome-Wide Association Studies*. Retrieved from http://www.genome.gov/20019523

National Human Genome Research Institute. (2014j). *Human Genetic Variation*. Retrieved from http://www.genome.gov/27528712

National Human Genome Research Institute. (2014k). Messenger RNA. *Talking Glossary of Genetic Terms*. Retrieved from http://www.genome.gov/glossary/index.cfm?id=123

National Human Genome Research Institute, (2014l). Pedigree. *Talking Glossary of Genetic Terms*. Retrieved from http://www.genome.gov/Glossary/index.cfm?id=148

National Human Genome Research Institute. (2014m). RNA. *Talking Glossary of Genetic Terms*. Retrieved from http://www.genome.gov/glossary/index.cfm?id=180

National Human Genome Research Institute. (2014n). Specfic Genetic Disorders. Learning about Cystic Fibrosis. Retrieved from http://www.genome.gov/10001213

Patrinos, G. P., Baker, D. J., Al-Mulla, F., Vasiliou, V., & Cooper, D. N. (2013). Genetic tests obtainable through pharmacies: The good, the bad, and the ugly. *Human Genomics, 7*(17), 1–4. doi: 10.1186/1479-7364-7-17

Paulik, A., Grim, J., & Filip, S. (2012). Predictors of irinotecan toxicity and efficacy in treatment of metastatic colorectal cancer. *Acta Medica (Hradec Kralove), 55*(4), 153–159.

Pharmacogenomics Knowledge Implementation. (2014). CPIC: Clinical pharmacogenetics implementation consortium. Retrieved from http://www.pharmgkb.org/page/cpic.

Phillips, E. J. Chung, W-H., Mockenhaupt, M., Roujeau, J-C., & Mallal, S.A. (2011). Drug hypersensitivity: Pharmacogeneticsw and clinical syndromes. *Journal of Allergy and Clinical Immunolology, 127*(3 Suppl), S60–S66. doi: 10.1016/j.jaci.2010.11.046

Price, M. J. (2012). Genetic considerations. *Advances in Cardiology, 47,* 100–113. doi: 10.1159/000338043

Savard, M., Dupré, N., & Brunet, D. (2013). Propofol-related infusion syndrome heralding a mitochondrial disease: Case report. *Neurology, 81*(8), 770–771.

Shao, H., Li, J., Zhou, Y., Ge, Z., Fan, J., Shao, Z., & Zeng, Y. (2008). Dose-dependent protective effect of propofol against mitochondrial dysfunction in ischaemic/reperfused rat heart: role of cardiolipin. *British Journal of Pharmacology, 153*(8), 1641–1649.

Smith, R. S., Gutierrez-Arcels, M., Tran, C. W., Park, S., Couter, C. J., & Lee, C. (2008). *Structural Diversity of the Human Genome and Disease Susceptibility.* Retrieved from http://onlinelibrary.wiley.com/doi/10.1002/9780470015902.a0020764/full

Stepien, K. M., Tomaszewski, M., Tomaszewska, J., & Czuczwar, S. J. (2012). The multidrug transporter P-glycoprotein in pharmacoresistance to antiepileptic drugs. *Pharmacology Reports, 64*(5), 1011–1019.

United States Food and Drug Administration (FDA). (2008). Guidance for Industry. E15 Definitions for Genomic Biomarkers, Pharmacogenomics, Pharmacogenetics, Genomic Data and Sample Coding Categories. 2008. Retrieved from http://www.fda.gov/downloads/drugs/guidancecomplianceregulatory-information/guidances/ucm073162.pdf

United States Food and Drug Administration (FDA) (2014a). Highlights of (prasugrel) prescribing information. Retrieved from http://www.accessdata.fda.gov/drugsatfda_docs/label/2013/022307s010lbl.pdf

United States Food and Drug Administration (FDA) (2014b). Highlights of (ivacaftor) prescribing information. Retrieved from http://www.accessdata.fda.gov/drugsatfda_docs/label/2014/203188s008lbl.pdf

Ventola, C. L. (2011a). Pharmacogenomics in clinical practice: reality and expectations. *Pharmacology and Therapeutics, 36*(7), 412–450.

Ventola, C. L. (2011b). Direct-to-consumer pharmaceutical advertising: therapeutic or toxic? *Pharmacolgoy and Therapeutics, 36*(10), 669–684.

Yamazaki, H., & Shimizu, M. (2007). Genetic polymorphism of the flavin-containing monooxygenase 3 (FMO3) associated with trimethylaminuria (fish odor syndrome): observations from Japanese patients. *Current Drug Metabolism, 8*(5), 487–491.

Zolk, O. (2012). Disposition of metformin: variability due to polymorphisms of organic cation transporters. *Annals of Medicine, 44*(2), 119–129. doi: 10.3109/07853890.2010.549144

Genomic Technologies and Resources

Daniel Brazeau, PhD

2

The genomics revolution is, in many ways, a technological revolution that has provided scientists and clinicians with a battery of tools that provide the possibility of identifying the molecular mechanisms that underlie human disease. These tools thereby provide ways to reduce the risk as well as develop new potential drug targets or improve the ones we have. As is often the case with technological revolutions, advances in technology have far exceeded our ability to comprehend the massive amounts of data now being generated. Indeed, the ability to generate sequence data far exceeds our ability to analyze the data. The field of bioinformatics—often referred to as Big Data—has grown to address the deficiencies in data handling, annotation, and statistics of the immense datasets being generated from these next-generation sequencing technologies. Unfortunately, our extremely rudimentary knowledge of life's complexities at the molecular level greatly hampers our ability to apply these data to modern healthcare. Hopefully, continued work will provide the understanding needed to unravel the nature of medical therapeutics and the diseases that trouble humankind.

The ultimate identification and delineation of variants in human populations are critical to understanding the underlying genetic causes of human disease and drug response. The goal of this chapter is to provide the reader with a modest working

OBJECTIVES

- Discuss the role that technological advances in molecular biology have had in modern healthcare.
- Discuss the clinical applications of next-generation DNA sequencing.
- List, compare, and contrast the main genomic and pharmacogenomic databases.
- Introduce educational materials designed for individuals in the healthcare profession to stay up-to-date on the growing body of genomic information.

knowledge of the technologies involved in order to assess the significance and limitations of this research in its application to clinical practice.

Advances in Molecular Biology

A little over a decade has passed since the publication of the initial draft of the human genome (Lander et al., 2001; Venter et al., 2001). That effort took approximately 5 years and cost 2.7 billion dollars. As next-generation sequencing (NGS) technologies became available, the cost has decreased and sequence yields increased exponentially. Data from the U.S. National Human Genome Research Institute (NHGRI) Genome Sequencing Program (www.genome.gov/sequencingcosts) shows that the cost of obtaining a human genome in April 2010 was estimated at $31,125. This represents an $800,000 cost reduction per genome (Data from the NHGRI Genome Sequencing Program, http://www.genome.gov/sequencingcosts). As of April, 2014, the cost per genome was $4,920, which shows a sixfold reduction in 4 years. The goal of the NHGRI is to sequence a human genome for $1,000. Similarly, the time required to sequence the human genome has gone from 5 years in 2001 to weeks in 2013.

The ability to determine the sequence of a given DNA strand was first described by Sanger (Sanger, Nicklen, & Coulson, 1977). The Sanger "dideoxy" method for sequencing took advantage of the fact that special nucleotides (dideoxynucleotide triphosphates, or ddNTPs), when incorporated into a growing DNA strand, stop the continued addition of more nucleotides to the strand. Thus, a single DNA strand was "sequenced by synthesis" in four separate test tubes, each with a different chain terminating ddNTP. The DNA fragments generated in each tube could then be separated by size using polyacrylamide gels capable of distinguishing DNA fragments differing in length by a single base.

By the late 1980s, this process was automated; however, sequencing yields were limited by the number of sequencing reactions that could be performed. Typically, in automated systems, 96 reactions could be accomplished in 4 hours, each reaction generating 500–1000 base pairs of sequence. Thus, a single 4-hour run could generate as much as 96,000 base pairs of sequence data. Given a human genome of 3 billion base pairs, this would require more than 31,000 sequencing reactions (5,200 days) to sequence the genome once. This was the technology employed to sequence the first human genome. Clearly, new technologies employing new methodologies were needed to realize the genomic revolution.

Enzymes to Manipulate DNA

One of the key discoveries that initiated the revolution in molecular biology—and later, genomics—was the discovery of the cellular enzymes in bacteria that allowed researchers to cut or restrict DNA at specific sites, thus generating workable small fragments.

Although the ability to isolate relatively pure DNA has been available for more than 100 years, difficulties arise in how one might cut the DNA into small fragments with precision. The genome is massive, and with the discovery of restriction *endonucleases* (restriction enzymes), the ability to reliably and repeatedly cut DNA at specific locations and recover specific fragments with known sequences at each end proved to be the breakthrough that allowed for the isolation and retrieval of specific DNA sections from the genome. This discovery fueled early initial studies and the cloning of DNA.

Polymerase Chain Reactions

Another equally crucial advance in molecular biology came with the discovery of a method to amplify a specific DNA fragment a billion-fold within a heterogeneous mix of DNA. The polymerase chain reaction (PCR) employs two short-specific DNA sequences (primers) that anneal to the opposing strands of denatured double-stranded DNA. The primer sequences are designed to flank the region of DNA that one wishes to amplify for further study. A thermostable DNA polymerase is used to synthesize new DNA strands complementary to the target strands. This synthesis step is repeated 20 to 40 times; each time the amount of target DNA is roughly doubled. In this way, one can isolate and amplify a specific piece of DNA from a complex genome in a few hours or less. This technology allows one to isolate, amplify, and clone any section of DNA of interest in the genome.

With the use of DNA dyes (SYBR Green I) or fluorogenic probes, the amount of DNA accumulating with each cycle of the PCR amplification process can be quantified. Monitoring DNA quantities in real time allows researchers to estimate the initial starting concentration of a given target based upon the amplification profiles. From tissue samples as small as a few hundred cells, it is possible to estimate the number of messenger RNAs (mRNAs) present for any given gene of interest. Since mRNAs represent the first step in the pathway from the genome to the synthesis of cellular machinery, it is possible to assess the cellular response to a disease state or therapeutic treatment.

Real-time (or quantitative) PCR is also used to conduct genetic tests because the technique is sensitive enough to detect whether a patient carries one or two copies of any given single nucleotide polymorphism (SNP). The major limitation to using PCR is that one can evaluate only a single gene or SNP at a time. To understand the nature of disease or drug response, we need to be able to explore how the entire genome interacts, which requires a methodology that can assess the activity of many thousands of genes at the same time—and this has become possible only with the advent of advanced, or next-generation sequencing, technologies.

Next-Generation Sequencing

Recent next-generation sequencing (NGS) systems employ a number of slightly different strategies. Common to all is a methodology that immobilizes the DNA to be sequenced to a solid substrate, allowing for the individual amplification of the target DNA and the simultaneous sequencing of many thousands to billions of DNA strands in a single run (massively parallel sequencing; Ansorge, 2009; Metzker, 2010).

These emerging NGS technologies have reduced the time required to sequence a human genome from years to nearly days. More importantly, the cost and speed of genome sequencing have reached levels comparable to many standard medical tests. The ability to sequence a patient's entire genome—or a patient's tumor genome—is the basis of the genome revolution (Aparicio & Huntsman, 2010; Tucker, Marra, & Friedman, 2009; Voelkerding, Dames, & Durtschi, 2009). As noted earlier herein, the major limitation to using these technologies is our lack of knowledge of the relationship between genetic data and human health.

Given the decreasing cost of sequencing human genomes, an effort is underway to sequence sparsely the genomes of 1,000 individuals (the 1000 Genomes Project, www.1000genomes.org/) in order to identify SNPs and insertion/deletion variants in human populations (at least those with frequencies of 1%). As noted earlier, one of the fundamental goals of personalized medicine is the ultimate identification and delineation of the variants in human populations that are critical to understanding the underlying genetic causes of human disease and drug response.

Another equally exciting area where NGS has had impact is in studies of gene expression (Wang, Gerstein, & Snyder, 2009). These studies typically assess which genes are *up-regulated* (turned on or increased in expression) or *down–regulated* (turned off or reduced in expression) in the course of disease progression or in response to therapeutic treatment. Typically, such studies involve the collection of mRNAs from tissue samples or cells of interest and then quantifying the mRNAs that have increased or decreased in abundance compared with control samples. NGS, with its massively parallel sequencing, allows for the sequencing of the entire mRNA pool (RNA Seq) within a sample. With this technology, known genes (mRNAs) are quantified and previously unknown transcripts are discovered.

A slight variation on RNA Seq is whole exome sequencing (WES). An estimated 85% of the disease-causing mutations occur in coding regions of the genome (Botstein & Risch, 2003). The *exome* is that portion of the human genome that directly encodes proteins. In the genome are approximately 180,000 exons (DNA sequences within a gene that are transcribed into the mRNA), making up about 1% of the human genome. WES uses NGS technologies to sequence most of the exomes in an individual—approximately 30 million base pairs. As is the case in the 1000 Genome Project, WES seeks to identify the genetic variation among patients present in the exome. Mutations in these sequences are much more likely to have severe consequences than in the remaining 99% of the human genome. The goal of this approach is to identify genetic variation that is responsible for common diseases, such as cystic fibrosis, autism, and Alzheimer's disease, without the high expenses incurred in sequencing the entire genome (Rabbani, Tekin, & Mahdieh, 2014).

NGS is quickly becoming a cost-effective tool in many clinical settings. Sequence data, whether of the patient, the patient's tumor, or the mRNA pool of either, is now becoming readily available to aid clinicians in the diagnosis and treatment of diseases. Following are two specific examples of the application of NGS to healthcare.

Diagnosis of Genetic Disorders

Any given trait, such as height or disease state, is the result of the interaction between an individual's genetic makeup and environmental factors (diet, exposure to carcinogens, etc.). An individual's *genotype* describes the genetic component of a trait. The *phenotype* represents the outcome of the interplay of the genotype and environmental factors. Understanding genetic disorders is at the most basic level an understanding of the relationship of genotype to phenotype. In many cases, diseases that are phenotypically very similar to one another may have very different genetic causes. Often the genetic heterogeneity underlying the disease is unknown at presentation. Attempts to determine the genetic factors involved gene-by-gene would require many tests and much time, perhaps delaying treatment. For example, congenital muscular dystrophies include a group of genetic diseases involving at least 12 genes (North, 2008). Mutations in one or more of these genes may result in changes in biochemical or cellular pathways that result in similar structural changes in muscles producing the same outward pathology. NGS tests allow for the simultaneous assessment of the genetic makeup for 25 genes involved in these pathways to quickly identify the specific genetic cause and potentially guide therapy (Jones et al., 2011).

Pharmacogenomics in Action

Lynch syndrome—often called *hereditary nonpolyposis colorectal cancer*—is an inherited disorder that increases the risk of many types of cancer, particularly cancers of the colon (large intestine) and rectum. Many of the genes associated with Lynch syndrome are involved in the repair of mistakes that occur during DNA synthesis, which is a normal step in cell division. Often these mutations are inherited in an autosomal dominant pattern. Differentiating is often difficult among the possible genetic disorders based upon clinical guidelines. NGS tests (panels), however, are now available to test simultaneously for mutations in many of these "repair" genes. This information allows for a more accurate diagnosis based on the underlying cause rather than general disease presentation. The ultimate goal is to treat the underlying cause rather than treat symptoms.

Mitochondrial disorders represent the most common form of metabolic disorders. Even though the mitochondrial genome is minute compared with the nuclear genome (greater than 40,000 times smaller), mitochondrial disorders generally have diverse presentations because underlying causative mutations may occur in the mitochondria or in nuclear genes that interact with the mitochondria (Wong, 2013). This complex set of clinical presentations makes diagnosis very difficult, expensive, and time-consuming. NGS panels allow for the testing of the entire mitochondrial genome and the many nuclear genes. In one study, a mitochondrial gene panel that included 1,000 nuclear genes was used to examine 42 infants suspected of suffering from mitochondrial oxidative phosphorylation disorders. Fifty-five percent of the infants were found to have mutations in the genes examined, and 24% in genes previously linked to disease (Vasta, Ng, Turner, Shendure, & Hahn, 2009).

Noninvasive Prenatal Diagnosis

Prenatal diagnosis is a critical component of modern healthcare practice. The trend in modern societies has been one of increasing maternal age for pregnancies, resulting in increased risk of fetal chromosomal abnormalities. Invasive techniques, such as amniocentesis and chronic villus sampling, carry significant risk—~1% miscarriage—limiting their use to high-risk pregnancies. Noninvasive prenatal genetic diagnosis based upon using maternal peripheral blood takes advantage of the fact that within maternal blood circulates fetal genetic material in the form of fetal cells and cell-free fetal DNA. The amount of material from either source is highly variable, and enrichment techniques of this DNA have had low efficiency to date. However, techniques are improving; and the hope is that very soon, a simple blood draw from the mother will allow clinicians to assess the genetics of the fetus.

To date, most significant advances have been in the fetal NGS analyses of trisomies involving the 21st, 18th, and 13th chromosomes (Valencia, Pervaiz, Husami, Qian, & Zhang, 2013). These techniques have been successful, using DNA extracted from maternal plasma (Chiu et al., 2008, 2011). In addition, the discovery of cell-free fetal DNA in maternal plasma (Lo et al., 1997) has made possible the analysis of at least the paternal component of the child's genome (fetal sex, RhD blood group, some single gene genetic disorders). Sinuhe, Lapaire, Tercanli, Kolla, & Hösli (2011) offer an excellent review of the present limitations and possibilities.

Genomic and Pharmacogenomic Databases

As noted, one of the most daunting issues arising from advancing technologies is the massive amount of data and information that is accumulating, including information concerning:

- Tissue-specific gene expression patterns for many diseases, particularly cancers
- Tumor sequence data for diagnosis and guidance of therapy
- Sequence data related to the genetic basis of many diseases
- Specific mutations that play a role in drug response: that is, pharmacogenetics

The amount of information is both massive and constantly increasing. The very best source for timely knowledge concerning the genetics of human health are the databases accessible via the Internet. As might be expected given the sheer size of the Internet, a great many websites provide genomic and pharmacogenomic information. Two databases with the most comprehensive, up-to-date, and trustworthy genomic or pharmacogenomic data are the National Center for Biotechnology Information (NCBI; www.ncbi. nlm.nih.gov/) and the Pharmacogenomics and Pharmacogenetics Knowledge Base (www. pharmgkb.org/). Both databases include primary data and literature as well as annotated databases. Both databases are free to the public, offering helpful online tutorials and glossaries for navigating through the immense databases.

The National Center for Biotechnology Information

The NCBI at the National Institutes of Health (NIH) was created in 1988 as the ultimate repository for all molecular biology information (Sayers et al., 2010). Likely, the largest portion of the NCBI database is GenBank (www.ncbi.nlm.nih.gov/genbank/), which is the repository for DNA sequence data from around the world (in collaboration with the European Molecular Biology Laboratory [EMBL] and the DNA Database of Japan [DDBJ]). NCBI is also responsible for the collection and dissemination of many other forms of molecular and genetic data, including protein sequences, taxonomic data, structural data, scientific literature, and the SNP database, to name only a few.

The NCBI has a highly integrated search and retrieval system—Entrez—that links all the databases. Entrez allows for the quick movement from one database to another within NCBI. With a simple mouse click, users can quickly go from an examination of a given mRNA sequence (GenBank) to identifying that sequence's location within the genome (Genome database) to information about that gene's role in human disease to its three-dimensional structure (3D Structures database) to the literature (PubMed).

The database most relevant to human disease, drugs, and genetics is the Online Mendelian Inheritance in Man (OMIM). The OMIM database is the repository for all data concerning human genes and genetic diseases. It has textual information and references with links to MEDLINE and all the many additional related resources at NCBI, including sequence data, genetic maps, and SNP data. OMIM is searchable by disease name, gene name, or drug name. As of 2010, the database has records for more than 13,161 human genes. Linked to OMIM is a free database (ClinVar) that collects and disseminates information regarding the relationships among human genetic variation and clinical phenotypes.

The Pharmacogenomics and Pharmacogenetics Knowledge Base

The Pharmacogenomics and Pharmacogenetics Knowledge Base (PharmGKB) is an integrated database providing clinical, pharmacokinetic, pharmacodynamic, genotypic, and molecular function data for human genetic polymorphisms and drugs (Altman et al., 2003; Klein et al., 2001). PharmGKB is the absolute best source for up-to-date information concerning genes and drug response. The stated aim of this database developed and maintained by Stanford University is to "aid researchers in understanding how genetic variation among individuals contributes to differences in reactions to drugs." The data within PharmGKB includes:

- Annotation of genetic variants that play a role in gene-drug-disease relationships
- Excellent summaries of important *pharmacogenes* (genes involved in drug response)
- FDA drug labels that include pharmacogenomic information
- Drug metabolism and transport pathways with links to relevant genes
- Clinical annotations summarizing the role of human genetic variation in altering clinical endpoints that aid in determining medical practice or policy
- Published pharmacogenomic drug dosing guidelines through the Clinical Pharmacogenetics Implementation Consortium (CPIC)

The PharmGKB collects, curates, and makes available to all health professions knowledge concerning human genetic variation and drug response. Similar to the NCBI database, PharmGKB includes helpful tutorials on how to navigate the database.

Additional Online Resources

The pace of genomic information growth makes the NCBI and PharmGKB indispensable resources for up-to-date pharmacogenomic information. All healthcare professionals should be familiar with the use of these repositories of genetic information. Additionally, a number of web-based resources provide educational materials specifically designed for individuals in the healthcare profession. These include the following excellent sites:

- **Global Genetics and Genomics Community (G3C)(http://g-3-c.org/en):** An educational resource that presents case studies demonstrating how genetics influences human health and illness through genomic healthcare simulations

- **Wellcome Trust Sanger Institute's Your Genome (www.yourgenome.org/):** An educational resource designed to help the public understand the role of genetics and genomic science in human health
- **National Coalition for Health Professional Education in Genetics (NCHPEG.org):** Promotes health professional education about advances in human genetics
- **Pharmacogenomics Education Program (https://pharmacogenomics.ucsd. edu/):** Program for healthcare professionals to increase awareness of the utility of pharmacogenomics, pharmacogenomic tests, and their therapeutic use

Summary

The availability of diagnostic tests based upon NGS technologies will provide:

- Opportunities to identify patients early in life with potential health issues
- Elimination of lengthy and often invasive procedures by correctly identifying the under-causative agent
- Aid in the development of new lifesaving therapies
- Permitting prompt management and accurate genetic counseling

Furthermore, the ability to diagnose patients quickly and accurately will stimulate the development of targeted therapies based on the known genetic defects. The analysis of genetic data from patients with uncharacterized molecular defects will allow the discovery of novel mutations in the targeted candidate genes.

Questions

What are restriction endonucleases? Why are these enzymes so crucial to the development of molecular biology and genomics?

What are some of the clinical implications of next-generation sequencing technologies?

What are the differences between PCR and real-time PCR?

What are the differences between whole genome sequencing and whole exome sequencing?

What resources are available at PharmGKB?

References

Altman, R. B., Flockhart, D. A., Sherry, S. T., Oliver, D. E., Rubin, D. L., & Klein, T. E. (2003). Indexing pharmacogenetic knowledge on the World Wide Web. Pharmacogenetics, 13, 3–5.

Ansorge, W. J. (2009). Next-generation DNA sequencing techniques. N Biotechnology, 25, 195–203.

Aparicio, S. A., & Huntsman, D. G. (2010). Does massively parallel DNA resequencing signify the end of histopathology as we know it? *The Journal of Pathology, 220*, 307–315.

Botstein, D., & Risch, N. (2003). Discovering genotypes underlying human phenotypes: past successes for Mendelian disease, future approaches for complex disease. *Nature Genetics, 33*(Suppl), 228–237.

Chiu, R. W., Akolekar, R., Zheng, Y. W., Leung, T. Y., Sun, H., Chan, K. C., . . . Lo, Y. M. (2011). Non-invasive prenatal assessment of trisomy 21 by multiplexed maternal plasma DNA sequencing: large-scale validity study. *The BMJ, 342*, c7401.

Chiu, R. W., Chan, K. C., Gao, Y., Lau, V. Y., Zheng, W., Leung, T. Y., . . . Lo, Y.M. (2008). Noninvasive pre-natal diagnosis of fetal chromosomal aneuploidy by massively parallel genomic sequencing of DNA in maternal plasma. *Proceedings of the National Academy of Sciences, 105*(51), 20458–63.

Jones, M. A., Bhide, S., Chin, E., Ng, B. G., Rhodenizer, D., Zhang, V. W., . . . Hegde, M. R. (2011). Targeted polymerase chain reaction-based enrichment and next generation sequencing for diagnostic testing for congenital disorders of glycosylation. *Genetics of Medicine, 13*, 921–932.

Klein, T. E., Chang, J. T., Cho, M. K., Easton, K. L., Fergerson, R., Hewett, M., . . . Altman, R. B., (2001). Integrating genotype and phenotype information: an overview of the PharmGKB Project. *The Pharmacogenomics Journal, 1*, 167–170.

Lander, E. S., Linton, L. M., Birren, B., Nusbaum, C., Zody, M. C., Baldwin, J., . . . Wyman, D. (2001). Initial sequencing and analysis of the human genome. *Nature, 409*, 860–921.

Lo, Y. M., Corbetta, N., Chamberlain, P. F., Rai, V., Sargent, I. L., Redman, C. W. G., & Wainscoat, J. S. (1997). Presence of fetal DNA in maternal plasma and serum. *Lancet, 350*, 485–487.

Metzker, M. L. (2010). Sequencing technologies — the next generation. *Nature Review Genetics, 11*, 31–46.

North, K. (2008). What's new in congenital myopathies? *Neuromuscular Disorders, 18*(6), 433–442.

Rabbani, B., Tekin, M., & Mahdieh, N. (2014). The promise of whole-exome sequencing in medical genetics. *Journal of Human Genetics, 59*, 5–15.

Sanger, F., Nicklen, S., & Coulson, A. R. (1977). DNA sequencing with chain-terminating inhibitors. *Procedings of the National Academy of Sciences USA, 74*(12), 5463–5467.

Sayers, E. W., Barrett, T., Benson, D. A, Bryant, S. H., Canese, K., Chetvernin, V., . . . Ye, J. (2010). Database resources of the National Center for Biotechnology Information. *Nucleac Acids Research, 38*, D5–16.

Sinuhe, H., Lapaire, O., Tercanli, S., Kolla, V., & Hösli, I. (2011). Determination of fetal chromosome aberra-tions from fetal DNA in maternal blood: has the challenge finally been met? *Expert Reviews in Molecular Medicine, 13*, e16.

Tucker, T., Marra, M., & Friedman, J. M. (2009). Massively parallel sequencing: the next big thing in genetic medicine. *American Journal of Human Genetics, 85,* 142–154.

Valencia, C. A., Pervaiz, M. A., Husami, A., Qian, Y., & Zhang, K. (2013). Next-Generation-Sequencing based noninvasive prenatal diagnosis. In *Next generation sequencing technologies in medical genetics* (pp. 45-55). New York, NY: Springer.

Vasta, V., Ng, S. B., Turner, E. H., Shendure, J., & Hahn, S. H. (2009). Next generation sequence analysis for mitochondrial disorders. *Genome Medicine, 1*(10), 100.

Venter, J. C., Adams, M. D., Myers, E. W., Li, P. W., Mural, R. J., Sutton, G. G., . . . Zhu, X. (2001). The sequence of the human genome. *Science, 291,* 1304–1351.

Voelkerding, K. V., Dames, S. A., & Durtschi, J. D. (2009). Next-generation sequencing: from basic research to diagnostics. *Clinical Chemistry, 55,* 641–658.

Wang, Z., Gerstein, M., & Snyder, M. (2009). RNA-Seq: a revolutionary tool for transcriptomics. *Nature Reviews Genetics, 10,* 57–63.

Wong, L. J. (2013). Next generation molecular diagnosis of mitochondrial disorders. *Mitochondrion, 13*(4), 379–387.

Basics of Pharmacogenetics

Daniel Brazeau, PhD

3

Pharmacogenetics—the study of the role of human genetic variation in determining individual drug response—has been an active area of research into the role that human genetics plays in drug safety and efficacy (Kalow, 2004). The basic premise of pharmacogenetics is that for any given drug, one or more genes that encode proteins determine the drug's probable safety and efficacy in an individual patient.

Generally, pharmacogenetics has been limited to the effects of one or a few genes on drug efficacy and safety. Within pharmacogenetics are three broad classes of genes that differ in how they interact with a given drug:

- **Drug-metabolizing pharmacogenetics:** Examines the role of human variation in genes that code for enzymes that are involved in the metabolism of the drug. Genes include those that code for Phase I or II metabolizing enzymes and may either activate an inactive compound (prodrug) into an active agent or inactivate an active drug to an inactive metabolite. Generally, drug metabolizing pharmacogenetics results in differences among patients in the pharmacokinetics of the drug.

- **Drug-transporter pharmacogenetics:** Examines the role of human variation in genes that code for membrane transporters that move drugs either into or out of cells. Similar to drug metabolizing genes,

OBJECTIVES

- Discuss the importance of environmental responses and their potential impact on pharmacogenetic studies of drug response and disposition.

- Discuss two critical properties of a drug that need to be present if pharmacogenetics is to play a key role in optimizing patient care for a specific therapeutic agent.

- Discuss the nature of pharmacogenetic issues that one may expect with a specific drug based upon knowledge of the mechanism of action, metabolic, or transport properties.

drug-transporter pharmacogenetics results in differences among patients in the pharmacokinetics of the drug.

- **Drug-target pharmacogenetics:** Examines the role of human variation in genes that code for the direct target of the drug or code for other proteins that are associated with the biochemical or regulatory pathway of the drug. Unlike the pharmacogenetics of genes involved in drug metabolism or drug transport, drug-target pharmacogenetics often results in differences in the pharmacodynamics of the drug.

Pharmacogenomics

The study of the genome-wide role of human variation in drug response is often used interchangeably with "pharmacogenetics" but is a broader term that includes pharmacogenetic effects and the application of genomic technologies in drug discovery, disposition, and function.

With knowledge of the specific genes and with information on the genetic variation among patients for these genes, adjusting dosages or suggesting alternative therapies that yield the best outcomes for the patient is possible. Extensive literature, including several new journals, details studies showing gene-drug relationships and the importance of including a patient's genetic makeup in guiding therapeutic decision-making (Efferth & Volm, 2005; Weinshilboum & Wang, 2004). Pharmacogenetics can play an important role in identifying responders and nonresponders to medications, thus avoiding adverse events and optimizing drug dosages. As of 2014, the FDA lists more than 140 drugs (see Table 3.1) for which there are molecular biomarkers that may aid in better therapeutic outcomes for patients carrying these genetic markers (www.fda.gov/drugs/sciencere-search/researchareas/pharmacogenetics). Biomarkers include markers that may be heritable or somatic gene variants, functional deficiencies, expression changes, and chromosomal abnormalities.

Table 3.1   FDA Pharmacogenomic Biomarkers in Drug Labeling

Therapeutic Area	Drug	Gene Name	FDA Labeling Sections
Analgesic/ Anesthesiology	Tramadol	CYP2D6	Clinical Pharmacology
	Codeine	CYP2D6	Boxed Warnings, Warnings and Precautions, Use in Specific Populations, Clinical Pharmacology, Patient Counseling Information
Autoimmune Diseases	Belimumab	BTG3	Clinical Pharmacology, Clinical Studies
Cardiology	Carvedilol	CYP2D6	Drug Interactions, Clinical Pharmacology
	Clopidogrel	CYP2C19	Boxed Warning, Dosage and Administration, Warnings and Precautions, Drug Interactions, Clinical Pharmacology
	Isosorbide and Hydralazine	NAT1-2	Clinical Pharmacology
	Metoprolol	CYP2D6	Precautions, Clinical Pharmacology
	Prasugrel	CYP2C19	Use in Specific Populations, Clinical Pharmacology, Clinical Studies
	Propafenone	CYP2D6	Clinical Pharmacology
	Propranolol	CYP2D6	Precautions, Drug Interactions, Clinical Pharmacology
	Quinidine	CYP2D6	Precautions
	Ticagrelor	CYP2C19	Clinical Studies
Cardiology or Hematology	Warfarin	PROC, CYP2C9, VKORC1	Warning and Precautions
Dermatology	Cevimeline	CYP2D6	Drug Interactions
	Dapsone	G6PD	Indications and Usage, Precautions, Adverse Reactions, Patient Counseling Information
	Fluorouracil	DPYD	Contraindications, Warnings, Patient Information
Endocrinology	Atorvastatin	LDLR	Indications and Usage, Dosage and Administration, Warnings and Precautions, Clinical Pharmacology, Clinical Studies

continues

Table 3.1   FDA Pharmacogenomic Biomarkers in Drug Labeling *(continued)*

Therapeutic Area	Drug	Gene Name	FDA Labeling Sections
	Chlorpropa-mide	G6PD	Precautions
	Glimepiride	G6PD	Warning and Precautions
	Glipizide	G6PD	Precautions
	Glyburide	G6PD	Precautions
	Lomitapide	LDLR	Indication and Usage, Adverse Reactions, Clinical Studies
	Mipomersen	LDLR	Indication and Usage, Clinical Studies, Use in Specific Populations
	Pravastatin	LDLR	Clinical Studies, Use in Specific Populations
	Rosuvastatin	LDLR	Indications and Usage, Dosage and Administration, Clinical Pharmacology, Clinical Studies
Gastroenterology	Dexlanso-prazole	CYP2C19, CYP1A2	Clinical Pharmacology, Drug Interactions
	Esomeprazole	CYP2C19	Drug Interactions, Clinical Pharmacology
	Lansoprazole	CYP2C19	Drug Interactions, Clinical Pharmacology
	Omeprazole	CYP2C19	Dosage and Administration, Warnings and Precautions, Drug Interactions
	Pantoprazole	CYP2C19	Clinical Pharmacology, Drug Interactions, Special Populations
	PEG-3350, Sodium Sulfate, Sodium Chloride, Potassium Chloride, Sodium Ascorbate, and Ascorbic Acid	G6PD	Warnings and Precautions

Therapeutic Area	Drug	Gene Name	FDA Labeling Sections
	Rabeprazole	CYP2C19	Drug Interactions, Clinical Pharmacology
	Metoclopramide	CYB5R1-4	Precautions
Genitourinary	Tolterodine	CYP2D6	Warnings and Precautions, Drug Interactions, Use in Specific Populations, Clinical Pharmacology
Hematology	Eltrombopag	F5, SERPINC1	Warnings and Precautions
	Lenalidomide	del (5q)	Boxed Warning, Indications and Usage, Clinical Studies, Patient Counseling
	Methylene Blue	G6PD	Precautions
	Succimer	G6PD	Clinical Pharmacology
Infectious Diseases	Abacavir	HLA-B	Boxed Warning, Contraindications, Warnings and Precautions, Patient Counseling Information
	Boceprevir	IFNL3	Clinical Pharmacology
	Chloroquine	G6PD	Precautions
	Dapsone	G6PD	Precautions, Adverse Reactions, Overdosage
	Mafenide	G6PD	Warnings, Adverse Reactions
	Maraviroc	CCR5	Indications and Usage, Warnings and Precautions, Clinical Pharmacology, Clinical Studies, Patient Counseling Information
	Nalidixic Acid	G6PD	Precautions, Adverse Reactions
	Nitrofurantoin	G6PD	Warnings, Adverse Reactions
	Peginterferon alfa-2b	IFNL3	Clinical Pharmacology
	Primaquine	G6PD	Warnings and Precautions, Adverse Reactions
	Quinine Sulfate	G6PD	Contraindications, Patient Counseling Information
	Rifampin, Isoniazid, and Pyrazinamide	NAT1-2	Adverse Reactions, Clinical Pharmacology

continues

Table 3.1   FDA Pharmacogenomic Biomarkers in Drug Labeling *(continued)*

Therapeutic Area	Drug	Gene Name	FDA Labeling Sections
	Simeprevir	IFNL3	Clinical studies, Clinical Pharmacology
	Sofosbuvir	IFNL3	Clinical Pharmacology, Clinical Studies
	Sulfamethox-azole and Trimethoprim	G6PD	Precautions
	Telaprevir	IFNL3	Clinical Pharmacology
	Terbinafine	CYP2D6	Drug Interactions
	Voriconazole	CYP2C19	Clinical Pharmacology, Drug Interactions
Metabolic Disorders	Carglumic Acid	NAGS	Indications and Usage, Warnings and Precautions, Special Populations, Clinical Pharmacology, Clinical Studies
	Velaglucerase Alfa	GBA	Indication and Usage, Description, Clinical Pharmacology, Clinical Studies
Neurology	Carbama-zepine	HLA-B, HLA-A	Boxed Warning, Warnings and Precautions
	Clobazam	CYP2C19	Clinical Pharmacology, Dosage and Administration, Use in Specific Populations
	Dextrome-thorphan and Quinidine	CYP2D6	Clinical Pharmacology, Warnings and Precautions, Drug Interactions
	Drospirenone and Ethinyl Estradiol	CYP2C19	Clinical Pharmacology, Warnings and Precautions, Drug Interactions
	Galantamine	CYP2D6	Special Populations
	Phenytoin	HLA-B	Warnings
	Tetrabenazine	CYP2D6	Dosage and Administration, Warnings, Clinical Pharmacology
	Valproic Acid	NAGS, CPS1, ASS1, OTC, ASL, ABL2, POLG	Boxed Warning, Contraindications, Warnings and Precautions

Therapeutic Area	Drug	Gene Name	FDA Labeling Sections
	Vortioxetine	CYP2D6	Dosage and Administration, Drug interactions, Clinical Pharmacology
Oncology	Ado-Trastuzumab Emtansine	ERBB2	Indications and Usage, Warnings and Precautions, Adverse Reactions, Clinical Pharmacology, Clinical Studies
	Afatinib	EGFR	Indications and Usage, Dosage and Administration, Adverse Reactions, Clinical Pharmacology, Clinical Studies, Patient Counseling Information
	Anastrozole	ESR1, PGR	Indications and Usage, Clinical Pharmacology, Clinical Studies
	Arsenic Trioxide	PML/RARA	Boxed Warning, Clinical Pharmacology, Indications and Usage, Warnings
	Bosutinib	BCR/ABL1	Indications and Usage, Adverse Reactions, Clinical Studies
	Brentuximab Vedotin	TNFRSF8	Indications and Usage, Description, Clinical Pharmacology
	Busulfan	Ph Chromosome	Clinical Studies
	Capecitabine	DPYD	Contraindications, Warnings and Precautions, Patient Information
	Cetuximab	EGFR, KRAS	Indications and Usage, Warnings and Precautions, Description, Clinical Pharmacology, Clinical Studies
	Cisplatin	TPMT	Clinical Pharmacology, Warnings, Precautions
	Crizotinib	ALK	Indications and Usage, Dosage and Administration, Drug Interactions, Warnings and Precautions, Adverse Reactions, Clinical Pharmacology, Clinical Studies
	Dabrafenib	BRAF, G6PD	Indications and Usage, Dosage and Administration, Warnings and Precautions, Clinical Pharmacology, Clinical Studies, Patient Counseling Information

continues

Table 3.1   FDA Pharmacogenomic Biomarkers in Drug Labeling *(continued)*

Therapeutic Area	Drug	Gene Name	FDA Labeling Sections
	Dasatinib	BCR/ABL1	Indications and Usage, Clinical Studies, Patient Counseling Information
	Denileukin Diftitox	IL2RA	Indications and Usage, Warnings and Precautions, Clinical Studies
	Erlotinib	EGFR	Clinical Pharmacology
	Everolimus	ERBB2, ESR1	Indications and Usage, Boxed Warning, Adverse Reactions, Use in Specific Populations, Clinical Pharmacology, Clinical Studies
	Exemestane	ESR1	Indications and Usage, Dosage and Administration, Clinical Studies, Clinical Pharmacology
	Fluorouracil	DPYD	Warnings
	Fulvestrant	ESR1	Indications and Usage, Clinical Pharmacology, Clinical Studies, Patient Counseling Information
	Ibritumomab Tiuxetan	MS4A1	Indications and Usage, Clinical Pharmacology, Description
	Imatinib	KIT, BCR/ABL1, PDGFRB, FIP1L1	Indications and Usage, Dosage and Administration, Clinical Pharmacology, Clinical Studies
	Irinotecan	UGT1A1	Dosage and Administration, Warnings, Clinical Pharmacology
	Lapatinib	ERBB2	Indications and Usage, Clinical Pharmacology, Patient Counseling Information
	Letrozole	ESR1, PGR	Indications and Usage, Adverse Reactions, Clinical Studies, Clinical Pharmacology
	Mercapto-purine	TPMT	Dosage and Administration, Contraindications, Precautions, Adverse Reactions, Clinical Pharmacology

Therapeutic Area	Drug	Gene Name	FDA Labeling Sections
	Nilotinib	BCR/ABL1, UGT1A1	Indications and Usage, Patient Counseling Information
	Obinutuzumab	MS4A1	Indication and Usage, Warnings and Precautions, Description, Clinical Pharmacology, Clinical Studies
	Ofatumumab	MS4A1	Indications and Usage, Clinical Pharmacology
	Omacetaxine	BCR/ABL1	Clinical Pharmacology
	Panitumumab	EGFR, KRAS	Indications and Usage, Warnings and Precautions, Clinical Pharmacology, Clinical Studies
	Pazopanib	UGT1A1	Clinical Pharmacology, Warnings and Precautions
	Pertuzumab	ERBB2	Indications and Usage, Warnings and Precautions, Adverse Reactions, Clinical Studies, Clinical Pharmacology
	Ponatinib	BCR-ABL T315I	Indications and Usage, Adverse Reactions, Clinical Pharmacology, Clinical Studies
	Rasburicase	G6PD	Boxed Warning, Contraindications
	Rituximab	MS4A1	Indication and Usage, Clinical Pharmacology, Description, Precautions
	Tamoxifen	ESR1, PGR, F5, F2	Indications and Usage, Precautions, Medication Guide
	Thioguanine	TPMT	Dosage and Administration, Precautions, Warnings
	Tositumomab	MS4A1	Indications and Usage, Clinical Pharmacology
	Trametinib	BRAF	Indications and Usage, Dosage and Administration, Adverse Reactions, Clinical Pharmacology, Clinical Studies, Patient Counseling Information
	Trastuzumab	ERBB2	Indications and Usage, Warnings and Precautions, Clinical Pharmacology, Clinical Studies

continues

Table 3.1   FDA Pharmacogenomic Biomarkers in Drug Labeling *(continued)*

Therapeutic Area	Drug	Gene Name	FDA Labeling Sections
	Tretinoin	PML/RARA	Clinical Studies, Indications and Usage, Warnings
	Vemurafenib	BRAF	Indications and Usage, Warning and Precautions, Clinical Pharmacology, Clinical Studies, Patient Counseling Information
Psychiatry	Amitriptyline	CYP2D6	Precautions
	Aripiprazole	CYP2D6	Clinical Pharmacology, Dosage and Administration
	Atomoxetine	CYP2D6	Dosage and Administration, Warnings and Precautions, Drug Interactions, Clinical Pharmacology
	Citalopram	CYP2C19, CYP2D6	Drug Interactions, Warnings
	Clomipramine	CYP2D6	Drug Interactions
	Clozapine	CYP2D6	Drug Interactions, Clinical Pharmacology
	Desipramine	CYP2D6	Drug Interactions
	Diazepam	CYP2C19	Drug Interactions, Clinical Pharmacology
	Doxepin	CYP2D6	Precautions
	Fluoxetine	CYP2D6	Warnings, Precautions, Clinical Pharmacology
	Fluvoxamine	CYP2D6	Drug Interactions
	Iloperidone	CYP2D6	Clinical Pharmacology, Dosage and Administration, Drug Interactions, Specific Populations, Warnings and Precautions
	Imipramine	CYP2D6	Drug Interactions
	Modafinil	CYP2D6	Drug Interactions
	Nefazodone	CYP2D6	Drug Interactions
	Nortriptyline	CYP2D6	Drug Interactions

Therapeutic Area	Drug	Gene Name	FDA Labeling Sections
	Paroxetine	CYP2D6	Clinical Pharmacology, Drug Interactions
	Perphenazine	CYP2D6	Clinical Pharmacology, Drug Interactions
	Pimozide	CYP2D6	Warnings, Precautions, Contraindications, Dosage and Administration
	Protriptyline	CYP2D6	Precautions
	Risperidone	CYP2D6	Drug Interactions, Clinical Pharmacology
	Thioridazine	CYP2D6	Precautions, Warnings, Contraindications
	Trimipramine	CYP2D6	Drug Interactions
	Venlafaxine	CYP2D6	Drug Interactions
Pulmonary	Indacaterol	UGT1A1	Clinical Pharmacology
	Ivacaftor	CFTR	Indications and Usage, Adverse Reactions, Use in Specific Populations, Clinical Pharmacology, Clinical Studies
Rheumatology	Azathioprine	TPMT	Dosage and Administration, Warnings and Precautions, Drug Interactions, Adverse Reactions, Clinical Pharmacology
Populations	Carisoprodol	CYP2C19	Clinical Pharmacology, Special
	Celecoxib	CYP2C9	Dosage and Administration, Drug Interactions, Use in Specific Populations, Clinical Pharmacology
	Flurbiprofen	CYP2C9	Clinical Pharmacology, Special Populations
	Pegloticase	G6PD	Contraindications, Patient Counseling Information
Transplantation	Mycophenolic Acid	HPRT1	Precautions, Environmental Factors and Drug Response

Environmental Factors and Drug Response

Before considering the role that the genetic makeup of a patient may play in our understanding of pharmacogenetics and drug response, it is essential to consider the influence of environmental factors in patient variation in drug response. Among geneticists or epidemiologists, environmental factors are all those determinants of a phenotype that are not genetic: that is, are not inherited. Examples would include diet, age, environmental exposures, other concomitant diseases, or other drugs being taken.

A great many environmental factors working alone or in concert determine how a given patient will respond to a drug (see Figure 3.1). With the advent of genomic technologies and knowledge, assessing the role an individual's genetic make-up or genotype plays in this response is becoming possible.

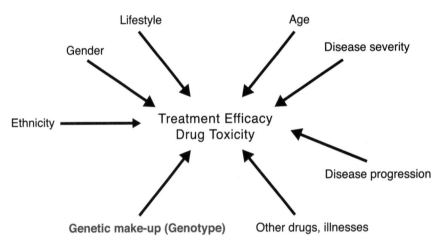

Figure 3.1   Environmental factors, including genetic makeup, influence treatment efficacy.

In many cases, the most important factors to consider are age, lifestyle, diet, and other concurrent drug therapies. Identifying the environmental factors involved in drug response is essential before the role of genetics can be accurately assessed. For example, many statins (HMG-CoA reductase inhibitors) taken to lower plasma cholesterol levels are known potent inhibitors of specific cytochrome P450 enzymes (Transon, Leeman, & Dayer, 1996). Specifically, the gene *CYP2D6* codes for the enzyme that is largely responsible for the conversion of codeine to morphine in the liver (see Figure 3.2). Codeine is a prodrug with little analgesic effect. It must be converted to morphine in the liver for pain relief. Patient outcome is dependent upon the type of mutation present in the gene *CYP2D6*.

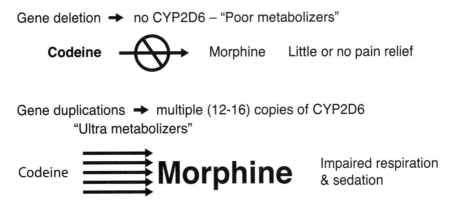

Figure 3.2   Codeine pharmacogenetics.

A polymorphism for this gene (referred to as the CYP2D6*4 allele), which is quite common in Caucasians, results in a nonfunctional phenotype. (See PharmGKB.org for the latest information on other variants and their frequencies in human populations.) Individuals *homozygous* (carrying this allele on both chromosomes) for this variant derive little or no pain relief upon taking codeine. Thus there is a clear genotype *(CYP2D6*4)*-to-phenotype (little or no analgesic response) relationship. However, the same phenotype (little or no analgesic response) may also be seen in patients who are taking statins for high cholesterol treatment. Similarly, ritonavir, a HIV-protease inhibitor, is a potent inhibitor of the metabolizing enzyme necessary for the metabolism of many statins. Thus, patients on concomitant therapy of a statin and ritonavir may exhibit toxicity (Chauvin, Drouot, Barrail-Tran, & Taburet, 2013) similar to that seen in patients who genetically lack active CYP3A, but the phenotype (poor response) is due to an environmental factor (ritonavir)—not genetics. It is crucial in the evaluation of any patient's response to therapy that environmental factors may often confound the relationship between genetics and a patient's given drug response.

Inherent Properties of "Pharmacogenetic" Drugs

In examining the documented cases of pharmacogenetic issues in patients, two basic elements are common. The first is inherent to the drug itself. Most drugs where pharmacogenetics is clinically relevant have a narrow therapeutic window. The appropriate therapeutic dosage (and blood concentration) range for these drugs is small; thus slight, genetically based differences in drug metabolism, absorption, distribution, or clearance may result in adverse effects in the patient. Drugs that have wide therapeutic windows, which show no adverse effects across a wide concentration range, are unlikely to have pharmacogenetic issues because most genetic differences in metabolism, absorption, or distribution will be within the range of the normally administered dose.

The second is inherent in the biological pathways involved in the drug's metabolism or transport. Often with drugs that have "pharmacogenetic" indications, a single gene (*monogenic*) principally controls at least one critical step in the drug response pathway. With a single gene influencing a critical step, genetics differences (*polymorphisms*) in this gene among patients may result in different patient outcomes. In contrast, drugs for which there are multiple alternate pathways or multiple genes (*polygenic*) involved are unlikely to elicit varying responses from polymorphisms in a single gene. Thus, most drugs that have pharmacogenetic indications have narrow therapeutic indices and have a critical step in their metabolism or transport controlled by a single gene.

Drug-Metabolizing Enzyme Pharmacogenetics

To examine some of the basic issues seen in pharmacogenetics, we will look in detail at three examples of the role pharmacogenetics plays in explaining variation in patient drug response. These examples involve drugs that have narrow therapeutic windows and have phenotypes that are determined by one or two genes. We will use these pharmacogenetic real-world examples to elucidate other features of both drugs and genetics that are important in understanding the limitations and complexities of pharmacogenetics in clinical use.

Pharmacogenetics of Codeine

Codeine is an opioid analgesic used for pain control, as a cough suppressant, and as an antidiarrheal. Codeine is a prodrug with little analgesic properties until converted into morphine in the liver (refer to Figure 3.2). This metabolic conversion is carried out by cytochrome P450 2D6 (CYP2D6). A great many genetic polymorphisms have been described for this gene in humans. A number of these polymorphisms (alleles CYP2D6 *4, *5, *6; for others, see PharmGKB.org) result in greatly reduced or no enzyme activity. Patients who carry two copies of these variant alleles (referred to as "poor metabolizers") have greatly reduced capacity to convert codeine into morphine, and therefore experience little analgesic effect from taking codeine. Importantly, in this case, there is no toxicity issue: rather, only a lack of efficacy. In contrast, some individuals carry more than two copies of this gene on one chromosome; in some cases, as many as 16 copies. Such individuals exhibit high levels of CYP2D6 activity and are characterized as "ultra-rapid metabolizers" of codeine. These individuals rapidly convert the standard dose of codeine into higher exposure to morphine, thus resulting in a higher risk of toxicity, including impaired respiration.

The "basics" to note:

- Codeine (and morphine) has very narrow therapeutic indices.
- Metabolism of codeine is dependent on a single gene (CYP2D6).
- Loss of function mutations (little or no active CYP2D6) in the metabolism of a prodrug generally results in loss of efficacy.
- Gain of function mutations (extra copies of CYP2D6) in the metabolism of a prodrug often results in toxicity from increased levels of the active metabolite (see Figure 3.3).

Drug Formulation	Gain-of-function Mutation	Typical or Wild Type Allele	Loss-of-function Mutation
	Increased Drug-Metabolizing Enzyme Activity	Normal Drug-Metabolizing Enzyme Activity	No Drug-Metabolizing Enzyme Activity
Active Drug	Little or No Active Drug	Appropriate Dose	Increased Active Drug Exposure
Pro Drug	Increased Active Drug Exposure	Appropriate Dose	Little or No Active Drug

Figure 3.3 Patient outcomes depending upon the nature of mutations in drug-metabolizing enzymes.

Pharmacogenetics of Thiopurine S-methyltransferase (TPMT)

Thiopurines are among the first line treatments for childhood acute lymphoblastic leukemia (ALL), organ transplant recipients, inflammatory bowel disease, and autoimmune diseases (Lennard, 1992). The enzyme thiopurine S-methyltransferase (TPMT) catalyzes the S-methylation of a number of chemotherapeutic prodrugs, such as 6-mercaptopurine (6-MP), 6-thioguanine (6-TG), and azathioprine (AZA). In the cell, 6-MP and AZA are converted into thioinosine monophosphate (TIMP) and ultimately to thioguanosine monophosphate (TGMP). TGMP is ultimately converted into cytotoxic nucleotide analogs (TGN), which inhibit DNA and RNA synthesis (see Figure 3.4). Of importance, 6-MP is a prodrug. The metabolism of 6-MP by TPMT is a critical step in the inactivation pathway leading to the ultimate clearance of the drug from the body.

Although a number of pathways are involved in the inactivation of these drugs, one gene (TPMT) is involved in the inactivation at each step (monogenic). That is, in each step of this activating pathway, the enzyme TPMT plays a role in inactivation. High concentrations of the cytotoxic nucleotide analogs (TGN) have been linked to hematopoietic toxicity and result in low patient tolerance to thiopurine therapies. Thus, loss of the drug inactivation pathways can have important clinical implications.

> Mercaptopurine (6-MP) is a prodrug requiring a number of enzymes for the production of the active compound TGN.

Clinically, polymorphisms in TPMT have been shown to play a role in explaining individual variation in response to thiopurine drug therapy. Low TPMT activity is associated with hematopoietic toxicity in patients treated with standard doses of 6-MP, 6-TG, or AZA (Krynetski & Evans, 1999; Weinshilboum & Sladek, 1980). Twenty-nine variant alleles in the gene TPMT have been identified in humans. The most common variant allele, TPMT*3A, is associated with low TPMT enzyme activity. Individuals carrying this allele on both chromosomes (homozygous) will experience extremely high concentrations of the active metabolite TGN with potentially fatal consequences. CPIC guidelines call for drastically reduced doses, 10-fold or less. Individuals with a single copy of the TPMT*3A allele and one normal allele (heterozygous) experience moderate concentrations of TGN and are advised to begin treatment with 30%–70% of the full dose.

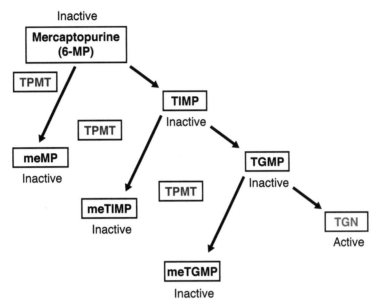

Figure 3.4   Pharmacogenetics of mercaptopurine.

The "basics" to note:

- 6-MP and its metabolites have very narrow therapeutic indices.
- The multiple inactivation pathways of these thiopurine drugs are largely dependent upon a single gene (TPMT).
- Reduced function mutations in TPMT result in toxicity from increased levels of the active metabolite (refer to Figure 3.4). This is the opposite outcome compared with the loss-of-function mutations in the codeine (a prodrug) example. Loss-of-function mutations in the inactivation pathways of active drugs often result in toxicity.

Pharmacogenetics of Warfarin

Warfarin is a commonly prescribed oral anticoagulant for the prevention and treatment of myocardial infarction, ischemic stroke, venous thrombosis, and atrial fibrillation. Warfarin is a very effective antagonist of the vitamin K epoxide reductase complex (VKORC1), which is a critical enzyme in the vitamin K-dependent clotting pathway (see

Figure 3.5). Warfarin is an active agent that inhibits Vitamin K reductase. Polymorphisms in the gene responsible for inactivation, CYP2C9, and the gene that encodes the direct drug target, VKORC1, will affect patient outcomes. Warfarin has a narrow therapeutic window with large interpatient variation. Insufficient drug concentrations may prevent thromboembolism. Overdosing may cause risk of bleeding events. Warfarin is delivered as a racemic mixture of the R and S stereoisomers. S-warfarin is the more potent inhibitor of VKORC1 by 3- to 5-fold and accounts for 60%–70% of the anticoagulation response. S-warfarin is largely metabolized by a single enzyme (CYP2C9) and thus behaves as a monogenic trait.

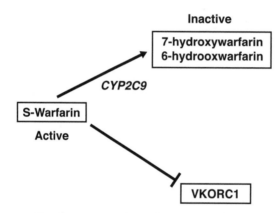

Figure 3.5   Warfarin pharmacogenetics.

To date, more than 50 variants in CYP2C9 have been described in human populations. Two variants, CYP2C9*2 and CYP2C9*3, are the most common. Patients with CYP2C9*2 and/or CYP2C9*3 variants metabolize warfarin slowly; thus, traditional dosing regimens may lead to bleeding events or longer times to achieve stable drug concentrations. Interestingly, the frequencies of CYP2C9*2 and CYP2C9*3 vary considerably among ethnic populations, with Caucasians having *2 and *3 frequencies from 8%–20% and 6%–10%, respectively. CYP2C9*2 and CYP2C9*3 are largely absent in Asian populations and are rare in African-American populations, with frequencies ranging from 1%–4%.

The "basics" to note:

- Warfarin has a narrow therapeutic index.
- The inactivation pathways of warfarin are largely dependent on a single gene (CYP2C9).
- Warfarin is an active drug and does not require activation via metabolism. Thus, loss of function or reduced function alleles in the gene involved in the inactivation pathway result in high exposure to the active compound and toxicity (refer to Figure 3.5).
- There is great variation among ethnic groups in the frequencies of the important alleles. Understanding the distribution of variant alleles among human populations is important to limit the universal application of single genetic tests if predicting drug response.

Drug-Transporter Pharmacogenetics

Transporters make up approximately 5% of proteins encoded within the genome. The genome of an organism encompasses all the genetic material in the cell. In humans, this would include the 3 billion base pairs contained in the chromosomes in the nucleus and the approximately 16,000 base pairs of the mitochondria.

Transporters are important in drug disposition and tissue penetration. Transporters mediate hepatobiliary, intestinal, and renal clearance and are the foundation of the blood-brain and placental barriers. Polymorphisms among humans in drug transporters may therefore result in differences among patients in drug disposition and clearance.

Generally, the pharmacogenetics of drug transporters presents a more complicated problem than that seen in the pharmacogenetics of drug-metabolizing enzymes. Unlike drug-metabolizing enzymes, whose basic function is independent of location, drug transporters may play different roles, depending upon the location of the transporters. For example, genetic differences in a transporter for an active drug may have different outcomes depending upon whether the transporter is in a hepatocyte (clearance) of the blood-brain barrier (possible toxicity). Thus, the literature describing the pharmacogenetics of drug transporters is often more complicated with outcomes dependent upon site of drug action or transport. Two examples of drug-transporter pharmacogenetics show this complexity.

Pharmacogenetics of Simvastatin

Simvastatin is a potent inhibitor of a coenzyme A reductase (HMG-CoA reductase), which is the rate-limiting enzyme in cholesterol biosynthesis. The Solute Carrier Organic Anion Transporter family member 1B1 (SLCO1B1) encodes a membrane-bound sodium independent organic anion-transporter protein (OAT1B1). This transporter plays an important function in mediating hepatic clearance of simvastatin. Two other members of this transporter family (SLCO2B1 and SLCO1B3) are also involved in the transport of statins (atorvastatin and lovastatin) into liver cells; however, the transport of simvastatin seems to be largely determined by SLCO1B1. Differences among patients in SLCO1B1 have been shown to result in differences in the pharmacokinetics of the drug. Individuals with loss of function or reduced function alleles exhibit a much higher exposure to active simvastatin (Pasanen, Neuvonen, Neuvonen, & Niemi, 2006), thus increasing the risk of myopathy. In these individuals, the CPIC recommends reduced dosing (http://www.pharmgkb.org/page/cpic).

The "basics" to note:

- The transport, and therefore clearance, of simvastatin is largely driven by a single gene, SLCO1B1. Other statins may have alternate transporters, and thus the same polymorphisms in SLCO1B1 that result in toxicity for simvastatin may have little effect for other statins.

- Simvastatin has a generally wide therapeutic index, and severe adverse reactions are relatively rare. However, the drug has pharmacogenetic indications because of the drug's high use resulting in a high number of actual cases of skeletal muscle toxicity (myopathy) and nonadherence.

Pharmacogenetics of P-glycoprotein

Many drugs are transported by the drug efflux pump (transporters that move compounds out of the cell) P-glycoprotein (P-gp). P-gp plays an important role in limiting drug bioavailability by effluxing them at the lumen-facing epithelia of the small intestine and colon, in elimination via biliary excretion, and in the proximal tubules in the kidney. P-gp also plays an important protective function because it restricts permeability of drugs and xenobiotics at the blood-brain, placental, and testis barriers.

More than 70 drugs are known substrates for P-gp, including antiepileptic and anti-tumor drugs. Assessment of P-gp expression has been correlated to treatment failure in epilepsy and to nonresponse in acute myeloid leukemia, childhood neuroblastoma, and other cancers (Ambudkar et al., 1999; Takara, Sakaeda, & Okumura, 2006). Differences in the expression of P-gp in a cell may result in resistance to the effects of a wide variety of drugs, and genetic variation in the expression of the protein may result in differing susceptibility to pharmacotherapy. The pharmacogenetic literature concerning P-gp and the gene that encodes it (ABCB1) is extensive, varied, and often contradictory, largely because of the many roles that this transporter plays in the body as well as the many compounds that interact with this transporter (environmental effects).

The "basics" to note:

- The pharmacogenetics of drug transporters is often complex. ABCB1, the gene that encodes P-gp, is a classic example of this complexity.
- P-gp is a substrate for many diverse drugs. The transporter is active at many sites throughout the body.
- P-gp function is also subject to induction or inhibition, depending upon the drug.

These factors make the pharmacogenetic indications for drugs transported by P-gp extremely complicated. The best source of information for the pharmacogenetics of P-gp (and ABCB1) can be found at PharmGKB.org.

Drug-Target Pharmacogenetics

In the same way that the genetic differences in the expression of genes that encode drug-metabolizing enzymes and drug transporters may influence patient response to a drug, genetic differences in the targets of the drug may also affect patient response. Included in drug-target pharmacogenetics are genes that encode direct protein targets of the drug, genes that encode downstream proteins in drug pathways including signal transduction pathways, and proteins involved in disease pathogenesis (Johnson & Lima, 2001). As noted earlier, drug-target pharmacogenetics often results in differences in the pharmacodynamics of response, resulting in loss of efficacy or resistance. This contrasts with the pharmacogenetics of genes involved in drug metabolism or drug transport, which alter drug pharmacokinetics.

Drug-target pharmacogenetics includes genes that encode receptors, transcription factors, and enzymes. We return to an earlier example, warfarin, to examine the role of genetic variation in drug targets and patient response. The target of warfarin is the vitamin K reductase enzyme. Vitamin K reductase is a key enzyme in the vitamin K recycling pathway. Vitamin K (in its reduced form) is important for a number of coagulation factors. Inhibition of vitamin K reductase by warfarin gives rise to the drug's anticoagulant properties. Vitamin K reductase is encoded by the gene VKORC1, for which there are at least five important variants and numerous less-common variants that contribute to inter-patient variation in warfarin dosing. The different allelic variants have different outcomes. Individuals with the VKORC1*2 variant require lower warfarin doses. This variant is common in Asians and Caucasians but rare in African populations (Geisen et al., 2005). The variants VKORC1*3 and VKORC1*4 require a higher warfarin dose. VKORC1*3 is the most common haplotype in African populations and is common in Caucasians.

The "basics" to note:

- Unlike the case for the pharmacogenetics of drug-metabolizing enzymes and drug transporters, the therapeutic index of the drug is often less important because genetic differences in drug targets generally result in differences in the pharmacodynamics of the drug: in this case, drug sensitivity or efficacy.
- Because we are considering the actual target of the drug, which is encoded by a single gene, we are by default talking about a monogenic trait.

Summary

Complexities are common to many pharmacogenetic drugs. In all cases, it is critical to remain aware of some of the basic attributes common to all pharmacogenetics:

- Unknown environmental factors may result in poor therapeutic outcomes (phenocopies) and may often mimic phenotypes caused by genetics.
- Drugs whose metabolism and transport are affected by multiple genes (*polygenic*) or multiple pathways do not generally exhibit pharmacogenetic indications.

- Drugs with wide therapeutic indices do not generally exhibit pharmacogenetic indications, though even "safe" drugs may have pharmacogenetic indications if they are widely prescribed.
- Clinically important genes often have many rare allelic variants with similar phenotypes.
- Variation in the frequencies of allelic variants among ethnic groups is very common. These differences in allelic frequencies may mask the role of any one variant, thus making single genetic tests less universal.

These issues are common to most gene/drug dynamics and do not preclude the importance of pharmacogenetic studies. What is necessary is a more basic understanding of the underlying factors common to all. Significantly, with an understanding of the genomic science underlying patient drug response and the ability to take advantage of resources, such as PharmGKB and National Center for Biotechnology Information (NCBI; www.ncbi.nlm.nih.gov), nurses and other healthcare providers will be better prepared to both use the genomic data now being collected and assimilate the new genomic discoveries to come.

Questions

What is meant by the statement *"The overall effects of medications are typically not monogenic traits"*? What does this mean in terms of phenotypic outcomes?

It has been said, *"An abnormal drug response that clusters within families provides strong evidence for a genetic cause."* Does this clustering provide sufficient proof?

How might allelic differences among populations or ethnic groups cause confusion in the application of pharmacogenetics in the clinic?

An understanding of pharmacogenetic factors influencing drug metabolism is important in understanding drug response and toxicity, at least for some narrow therapeutic range drugs. However, the pharmacogenetic differences in drug metabolism do not fully explain the variability observed in drug response. What are two factors that may contribute to the variability in drug response besides genetics?

References

Ambudkar, S. V., Dey, S., Hrycyna, C. A., Ramachandra, M., Pastan, I., & Gottesman, M. M. (1999). Biochemical, cellular, and pharmacological aspects of the multidrug transporter. *Annual Review of Pharmacology and Toxicology, 39,* 361–398.

Chauvin, B., Drouot, S., Barrail-Tran, A., & Taburet, A. M. (2013). Drug-drug interactions between HMG-CoA reductase inhibitors (statins) and antiviral protease inhibitors. *Clinical Pharmacokinetics, 52*(10), 815–831.

Efferth, T., & Volm, M. (2005). Pharmacogenetics for individualized cancer chemotherapy. *Pharmacology & Therapeutics, 107,* 155–176.

Geisen, C., Watzka, M., Sittinger, K., Steffens, M., Daugela, L. Seifried, E., . . . Oldenburg, J. (2005). VKORC1 haplotypes and their impact on the inter-individual and inter-ethnical variability of oral anti-coagulation. *Thrombosis and Haemostasis, 94,* 773–779.

Johnson, J., & Lima, J. J. (2001). Drug target pharmacogenetics. *American Journal of Pharmacogenomics, 1,* 271–281

Kalow, W. (2004). Human pharmacogenomics: the development of a science. *Human Genomics, 1,* 375–380.

Krynetski, E. Y., & Evans, W. E. (1999). Pharmacogenetics as a molecular basis for individualized drug therapy: the thiopurine S-methyltransferase paradigm. *Pharmaceutical Research, 16,* 342–349.

Lennard, L. (1992). The clinical pharmacology of 6-mercaptopurine. *European Journal of Clinical Pharmacology, 43,* 329–339.

Pasanen, M. K., Neuvonen, M., Neuvonen, P. J., & Niemi, M. (2006). SLCO1B1 polymorphism markedly affects the pharmacokinetics of simvastatin acid. *Pharmacogenetics and Genomics, 16*(12), 873–979.

Takara, K., Sakaeda, T., & Okumura, K. (2006). An update on overcoming MDR1-mediated multidrug resistance in cancer chemotherapy. *Current Pharmaceutical Design, 12*(3), 273–286.

Transon, C., Leeman, T., & Dayer, P. (1996). In vitro comparative inhibition profiles of major human drug metabolising cytochrome P450 isozymes (CYP2C9, CYP2D6 and CYP3A4) by HMG-CoA reductase inhibitors. *European Journal of Clinical Pharmacology, 50,* 201–215.

Weinshilboum, R. M., & Sladek, S. L. (1980). Mercaptopurine pharmacogenetics: monogenic inheritance of erythrocyte thiopurine methyltransferase activity. *The American Journal of Human Genetics, 32,* 651–662.

Weinshilboum, R. M., & Wang, L. (2004). Pharmacogenomics: bench to bedside. *Nature Reviews Drug Discovery, 3,* 739–748.

Integrating Pharmacogenomics Into Healthcare

Ellen Giarelli, EdD, RN, CRNP

4

At every level of practice, nurses will be involved in the application of pharmacogenomics to patient care (Guttmacher, Porteous, & McInerney, 2007). All nurses will need to know the difference between *pharmacogenetics* (the study of the role of inheritance in interindividual variation in drug response), and *pharmacogenomics* (the technology and knowledge base that analyzes how an individual's entire genetic makeup affects drug response; Becquemont, 2009). Nurses will need to know that pharmacogenomics deals with the influence of genetic variation on drug response in patients by correlating gene expression or single-nucleotide polymorphisms with a drug's efficacy or toxicity. They will need to apply their understanding that pharmacogenomics aims to develop rational means to optimize drug therapy, with respect to the patient's genotype, to ensure maximum efficacy with minimal adverse effects. Nurses, across services settings, will be part of practice and research that is driven by the promise of individualized drug therapy to maximize drug efficacy and minimize drug toxicity.

Science and technology have a way of leaping ahead of the readiness of clinicians to translate the science to patient care. The bench-to-bedside model challenges nurses to rise to a high level of practice with respect to pharmacogenomics. Are nurses ready for this challenge?

OBJECTIVES

- The bench-to-bedside model challenges nurses to integrate pharmacogenomics with practice
- Integrating pharmacogenomics in healthcare is guided by core competencies in genomics
- Pharmacogenomics provides information about genetic variation that will allow nurses to more carefully administer drugs

This chapter will discuss the roles and responsibilities of entry level and advanced practice nurses in the integration of pharmacogenomics with healthcare. The discussion will expand on the challenges faced by nurses as they endeavor to integrate pharmacogenomics with patient care and will propose that contemporary nursing education is producing nurses who will not be sufficiently prepared to take a significant role in bench-to-bedside pharmacogenomics.

Essential Competencies for Registered Nurses

Nursing faculty continually struggle to find a place in the undergraduate and graduate curricula for relevant content, emerging scientific evidence, and guidelines for efficient translation of findings to patient care. New knowledge competes for the limited time of students who, regardless of their education program (BSN to DNP), must demonstrate competence. With regard to genomics, a minimum expectation of a nurse graduate is that he or she has a basic understanding of genetics and genomics with regard to how these topics relate to and affect clinical practice. Our expectations for enhanced education of healthcare providers in genomics in general, and pharmacogenomics in particular, can be traced back nearly 20 years to the Human Genome Project (Collins, 1997). However, there has been little evaluation of such instruction and application to practice in nursing curriculum. Due to the competing demands of ever-increasing content, an apparent trend in undergraduate and graduate nursing curricula is to integrate genetics and genomics with course content, rather than teach them separately (Giarelli & Reiff, 2012).

In 2006 and 2012, the American Nurses Association defined the essential genetics and genomic competencies for all registered nurses and for advanced practice nurses, respectively (American Nurses Association, 2006; Greco, Tinley, & Siebert, 2011). These guidelines describe professional practice and professional responsibilities. These same guidelines may be translated to define and describe pharmacogenomics competencies. These competencies can be derived and generalized from specific uses of pharmacogenetic clinical exemplars. One exemplar is anticoagulant therapy.

One of the first widespread uses of pharmacogenetics is in prescribing the blood thinner warfarin (Coumadin). This drug has a narrow range of concentration in which it maintains acceptable anticoagulation and avoids adverse reactions. It is often prescribed for patients with cardiovascular disorders, such as atrial fibrillation, pulmonary embolism, and deep vein thrombosis (DVT). Management of warfarin therapy is generally complicated by the range of interaction effects with other medication (Marietta, Romero, & Malone, 2009). Individuals placed on this medication can have a 10-fold difference in the dose needed to be therapeutic. According to Lewis (2012, p. 395), a pharmacogenetic algorithm is available for use when prescribing warfarin.

In 2013, when nurses employed on a cardiac telemetry floor at a regional medical center on the East Coast of the United States were asked whether their patients were evaluated for the two variants in CYP2C9 and one variant of VKORC1, they admitted that they did not know anything about it. These nurses were graduates of a baccalaureate program and stated that one requirement was a course in pharmacology, and genetics was integrated with the curriculum.

Although the use of pharmacogenetic testing for these variants might be considered a standard of care by nurses in genetics, the actual testing is not at the standard conveyed to these nurse-teaching hospitals. Without data to support or refute, one might reasonably presume that "if there is one, there is another, someplace." Other institutions do not test for CYP2C and VKORC1 variants and employ nurses who have limited information on this practice.

Matching patients to drug therapy as a way to personalize medicine offers opportunities for practicing nurses to:

- Assist in the identification of patients who are likely to suffer an adverse reaction to a drug
- Help identify a drug most likely to be effective
- Help improve their focus and increase the efficiency of monitoring a patient's response to drug treatment
- Increase their capability to anticipate the course of an illness and prevent complications

These advantages must be integrated with the content of instruction in nursing education. All professions dealing with rapid change and scientific advancements face similar problems. Given that nurses are generalists, they must keep up with increasingly dense and new information and continually seek additional training to understand and interpret the value.

Pharmacogenomic Competency

In 1962, Brantl and Esslinger (1964) foretold genetic implications for the nursing curriculum. Ten years ago, Hetteberg and Prows (2004) reminded us of the passage of 40 years since the recommendation that genetics content be included in nursing curricula, and they offered a checklist for evaluating this process. Multiple articles describe the genetics content, the nurse training process, and achievement of expertise (Calzone et al., 2010, 2011; Calzone, Jenkins, Prows, & Masney, 2011; Daack-Hirsch, Dieter, & Quinn Griffin, 2011; Daack-Hirsch, Quinn Griffin, & Dieter, 2011; Greco, 2008; Greco, Tinley, & Seibert, 2011; Jenkins, Bednash, & Malone, 2011; Jenkins, Dimond, & Steinberg, 2001; Jenkins, Grady, & Collins, 2005a, 2005b; Jenkins & Lea, 2005; Lea, Feetham, & Monsen, 2001; Lea & Monsen, 2003; Lea, Skirton, Read, & Williams, 2011; Lewis, Calzone, & Jenkins, 2006). Genetics education has been labeled an ethical imperative (Kegley, 2003). There are ample resources to facilitate inclusion of genetics in nursing curricula and translation to practice, and the content has been delineated and parsed into the domains of nursing responsibilities and professional practice (National Institutes of Health/ National Human Genome Research Institute, 2014).

Competency Domains

Competency in genetics and genomics was recommended for all registered nurses by the American Association of Colleges of Nursing after deliberation at baccalaureate and master's education conferences (Calzone, Jenkins et al., 2011). Basically, competencies are grouped into two domains: professional responsibilities and professional practice. Professional responsibilities for the baccalaureate nurse include:

- Recognizing one's own attitudes and values related to genetics and genomic science
- Advocating for clients' access to desired services and resources
- Examining competency of practice on a regular basis, identifying areas of strength and need for professional development
- Incorporating genetic/genomic technologies and information with practice
- Demonstrating importance of tailoring care to the client's social and cultural profile
- Advocating for the rights of all clients for autonomous, informed genetic- and genomic-related decision-making (Calzone, Jenkins, Prows & Masny, 2011).

Each one of these responsibilities can be adapted to apply to pharmacogenomics.

The professional practice domain for the baccalaureate nurse is more extensive and prescriptive and includes four essential competency areas:

- Nursing assessment: applying/integrating genetic and genomic knowledge
- Identification
- Referral activities
- Provision of education, care, and support, each with one to eight specific areas of knowledge, and appropriate clinical performance indicators

Each of the essential competency areas further describes subcompetencies and for each of these, an area of knowledge specific to the subcompetency. In addition, clinical performance indicators are associated with each area of knowledge.

The complete list of essential competencies, subcompetencies, specific areas of knowledge, and corresponding clinical performance indicators can be found in Calzone and colleagues (2011) and can be viewed online at the Genetics and Genomics Competency Center for Education (G2C2, 2014).

Adapting a Core Competency

Nearly all the clinical performance indicators should be adapted to incorporate pharmacogenomics. One must first determine to what extent basic competencies are evident in nursing curricula. Teaching and promoting the application of core genetic/genomic competencies would naturally precede expansion of these competencies to pharmacogenomics.

People react differently to the same dose of the same drug because each person differs in the rates at which his or her body reacts to and metabolizes chemicals and medicines. With our growing understanding of the role of genetics in healthcare, there will be a growing need to develop tests to detect how variants of single or multiple genes affect drug metabolism and gene expression.

Risk assessment and interpretation of the relevance of risk-related data are basic components of advanced practice and will become components of basic nursing care in the future. As part of the process, nurses may be requesting diagnostic tests that help uncover genetic determinants of disease and helping patients to understand how these tests are interpreted. The two principal categories of testing will be pharmacogenetic tests and pharmacogenomic tests.

There are very specific ways that pharmacogenomics may be integrated with core competencies. Table 4.1 provides an example of how pharmacogenomics may be integrated with one specific competency in the professional practice domain and the essential competency of providing education, care, and support to clients with interpretation of selected genomic information or services.

Table 4.1 Integration of Pharmacogenomics with Nursing Genetic Core Competencies		
Specific Area of Knowledge	***Clinical Performance Indicator***	***Adapted Performance Indicator:***
Components of family history needed to identify disease susceptibility or genetic/genomic condition	Factors in a family and health history that contribute to: • Disease susceptibility • Disease characteristics • Treatment • Prognosis • Genetic/genomic condition • Response to treatment Use of family history information to inform health education	Discuss the interactive effect of factors in the family and health history of genetics in the selection of pharmacotherapeutics in treatment of disease, response to treatment, occurrence of side effects, and potential for adverse events during pharmacotherapy. Use family history on drug treatment response to inform health education and guidelines on communicating with healthcare providers and medication self-management.

Specific Area of Knowledge	Clinical Performance Indicator	Adapted Performance Indicator:
Inheritance patterns	The role of genetic, genomic, environmental, and psychosocial factors in the manifestation of disease	Discuss the interactive roles of pharmacogenetics, pharmacogenomics, environmental, and psychosocial factors in the response to treatment of disease.
Informed consent, procedures, and essential elements	Client's rights, ethical responsibilities of the nurse, and the balance of risks and benefits of treatments	Discuss the importance of offering testing for genetic variants prior to administering certain pharmacotherapeutics. Discuss the application of principles of privacy and confidentiality when consenting to genetic testing for a differential response to drugs.

Adapted from Calzone, Jenkins, Prows, & Masney (2011, p.188).

Adaption of the competencies requires systematic review of the overlap of pharmacogenetics and pharmacogenomics with each specific area of nursing knowledge and with the clinical performance indicators. A formal review and adaptation of the entire table of competencies will assure that the proposed integration becomes a fundamental part of nurse education and that nursing care will be informed by the most current literature and appropriately personalized to the patient's genetic profile. For the entire list of competencies and indicators for nurses, physician assistants, pharmacists, genetic counselors, and physicians, go to the Genetics and Genomics Competency Center for Education located at

www.g-2-c-2.org/start_search_map.php

The essential competencies in genetics and genomics for nurses with graduate degrees add to the core competencies and raise the level of responsibility and practice to match the expectation from all advanced practice nurses. There are 38 essential competencies in genetics and genomics for nurses with graduate degrees that are organized into categories of professional practice and professional responsibilities.

Professional practice for the nurse with a graduate degree defines and describes competencies of:

- Risk assessment and interpretation
- Genetic education, counseling, testing, and result interpretation
- Clinical management
- Ethical, legal, and social implications

Each of these competency areas has a list of associated behaviors to be demonstrated by the advanced practice nurse.

The professional responsibilities expected of the graduate nurse with regard to genetics include professional role, leadership, and research (Greco, Tinley, & Seibert, 2011). This cohort of nurses will soon include those with a doctorate of nursing practice (DNP). Standards of competent practice will be correspondingly higher. DNPs will be expected to translate evidence from pharmacogenomic research to practice.

Clinical Management/Interpretations

When personalizing pharmacotherapy, nurses will need to consider several factors in addition to genetics that will mediate effectiveness, or cause variability in drug response. These factors include:

Age of the patient	Genetics
Comorbid medical and psychiatric disorders	Patient's ability to adhere to treatment
Diagnosis/disease state	Patient's ability to observe for side or adverse effects
Exposures to pollutants, tobacco use	Patient's ability to understand purpose of the treatment
Family history with diagnosis and drug treatment	Polypharmacy (drug-to-drug interaction, drug-plus-drug synergy)
Food-to-drug interactions	Pregnancy
Formulation	Race, ethnicity
Gender	Route of administration

An important factor that can be addressed during the expert care provided by advanced practice nurses is the patient's ability to adhere to treatment. Poor medication adherence accounts for 33%–39% of all medication-related hospital admissions and costs approximately $100 billion per year in the United States alone (Osterberg & Blaschke, 2005). Several predictors of poor adherence will need to be adapted to the care of patients receiving medicines tailored to the individual genetic profile. Predictors that may be especially important to address with this population are:

- Complexity of treatment
- Cognitive impairment
- Inadequate follow-up or discharge
- Patient's lack of belief in the treatment
- Patient's understanding of the role of genetics in health

Pharmacogenomics measures aspects of an individual's response to drug therapy. This knowledge provides information about genetic variation that will allow more careful selection of drug and dosage regimen. With this information, nurses can more accurately and comprehensively monitor a patient's response to treatment and communicate relevant observations to other healthcare professionals, including prescribers and suppliers of pharmacotherapeutics.

Challenges to Integration by Nurses

Several challenges must be overcome to achieve the worthy goal of integrating pharmacogenomics with nursing care. The system-level obstacles are difficult to change, but if done, will be instrumental in affecting patient-nurse level change. Four main challenges are:

- Limited time in densely packed nursing curricula
- Evolving complexity of the science
- Uncertainty of the relevance of genomes to pharmacotherapy
- Limited funding for nursing research

Unless nursing curricula build in significant genetics content with nursing content, students will not be able to recognize the importance of genomics to patient care. When strong scientific evidence shows support of the value of pharmacogenomics testing and translation for patient care, there is good reason to feature such testing as part of the overall treatment plan. One way to accomplish this is to assure that basic genetic concepts are taught consistently and uniformly across school curricula.

Increase Time in Curricula for Genomics

A review of the content of baccalaureate nursing programs in the United States has uncovered a general inconsistency that may contribute to differences in nurses' knowledge of and application of genetic concepts to practice. Only 25% ($n = 191$) of the programs required a stand-alone course in genetics, while 75% had programs that integrated genetics content with other nursing content (Giarelli & Reiff, 2012). No data is available confirming that graduates of these programs are integrating their knowledge of genetics with patient care. However, based on the complexity and evolving nature of the science, one could argue the case for the need to include a course in basics genetics/genomic concepts as well as a curriculum with full integration of these concepts with principles of nursing care.

Opportunities to Learn Complexity of the Science

One significant challenge to integration is the evolving complexity of the science and its application. Many healthcare professionals were educated before the advent of pharmacogenomics, including nurses who graduated from any program prior to the onset of the Human Genome Project (1990) and, likely, until the human genome was sequenced and reported in 2003. Many, but not all, of these nurses are returning to earn their baccalaureate degrees. Unless these nurses returned to school in the last decade for advanced study, they may have little understanding of genetics and limited access to formal instruction. These nurses will need to learn the genomic vocabulary as it relates to treatment choices.

For example, few nurses may understand the clinical significance of the TATA box of the UGT1A1 gene (Nussbaum, McInnes, & Willard, 2007). For the nurse practicing in cancer care, it is important to know that polymorphisms of this gene contribute to an inherited variation in the toxicity of antineoplastics such as irinotecam (Camptosar; Innocenti & Ratain, 2004; Marsh & McLeon, 2004). This polymorphism and the polymorphisms affecting response to warfarin are noted in the FDA drug labels for these drugs. There are more than 50 pharmaceuticals with pharmacogenomic indications. This example illustrates the need for persistent continuing education, which may not be available to some or of interest to others.

The mandates for employers and advocates from within the nursing profession are to develop ways to provide continuing education without causing a financial or significant time burden to nurses and to stimulate their interest. Realizing either of these mandates will require considerable creativity.

Nurses may also not understand that variations in drug effects can be further classified as those due to either pharmacokinetic (drug metabolism, transport) or pharmacodynamic (drug targets) factors (Weinshilboum & Wang, 2004). These concepts must be understood along with the genetic concepts, such as gene-gene interactions, gene expression, polymorphisms, genotyping, and phenotyping. A relevant course in nursing curricula is pharmacology—and, ideally, pharmacogenomics. Furthermore, if nursing faculty do not possess a sophisticated understanding of these concepts, they will not be able to satisfactorily integrate them with nursing content.

> See Chapter 3 for coverage of drug-transporter and drug-target pharmacogenetics.

Decrease Uncertainty of Relevance

A challenge to preparing all nurses with knowledge of pharmacogenomics is their uncertainty of the relevance of genomics to general patient care. If a nurse believes that the content is relevant, he/she will be more likely to be interested in learning. One way to accomplish this is to demonstrate the relevance—using a simple illustration that, by developing a genetic profile with a positive predictive value for toxicity or an adverse reaction, nurses may be able to assure immediate and possibly long-term benefits for their patients. Minimally, nurses will satisfy an ethical obligation first to do no harm. The following examples illustrate this point.

Pain

A fundamental concept that crosses all areas of nursing care is pain. Nurses will believe the relevance of genetics if the pharmacogenomics of pain management is a thematic content strand. Nearly all patients will experience pain at some point, and all nurses must become experts in the assessment and treatment of pain.

Additionally, chronic pain management is a growing concern in the United States, and the use of opioids to treat pain (cancer- and noncancer-related) is a topic of discussion in the medical community and a contentious social issue when opiates are misused. The facts of addiction and efficacy make the use of opiates challenging, valuable, and controversial. Nurses monitoring patients' uses of pain medication track dosages and evaluate tolerance and side effects.

Substantial progress has been made in understanding how genetic variation can influence a patient's response to pain therapy, especially with regard to metabolic enzymes and opiate receptors (Stamer, Zhang, & Stuber, 2003). The majority of opioids used in pain management are metabolized by CYPs and/or UGT2B7 (Jannetto & Bratanow, 2009).

Nurses will prescribe codeine to patients across the lifespan. Codeine, for example, is converted in the liver by CYP2D6 to morphine. A person with the gene variant that causes poor metabolization of codeine will have less pain relief due to less availability of the metabolite (morphine). Without knowing this genetic difference, accurate dosing is unpredictable. The patient is unlikely to receive adequate analgesia from this drug (Snozek, Langman, & Dasqupta, 2012). Without pharmacogenomics testing, the prescribing physician and administering nurse may suspect a patient of drug diversion or exaggerating the level of perceived pain. Either assumption may lead to inappropriate and/or insensitive care. With pharmacogenomics testing and a comprehensive understanding of the variables and science, the nurse will be able to provide therapy and support, and accurately collect data from ongoing therapeutic drug monitoring.

Ethnicity and Race

Ethnic and racial differences in response to drug therapy are well known (Burroughs, Maxey, & Levy, 2002; Wilson et al., 2001). There is some evidence that these differences associate with genetic factors. Drug response is a complex trait and cannot be simply explained by describing differences among various racial groups in the frequencies of alleles involved in pharmacokinetic and pharmacodynamics components of drug therapy. According to Burchard et al. (2003), debate exists as to whether clinicians should include ethnicity and/or race as factors in decision making about drug choice. There is also debate and uncertainty as to the extent to which ethnic or racial groups are representative or inclusive of all or the majority. Cooper, Kaufman, and Ward (2003) posited that racial and ethnic labels are approximations and cannot be used to categorize or understand all members of the set. Geographic area may be as meaningful a label as ethnicity or race to organize information about medically relevant genetic differences.

> **NOTE**
>
> Nurses must be sensitive to the controversy associated with the role of ethnicity and race in personalized drug therapy while being open to consider the role of associated factors, such as environment, social experiences, diet, and potential effects of discrimination.

Racial disparities in blood pressure control have been well documented in the United States (Egan, Zhao, & Axon, 2010). Consistent findings show that Black Americans have high rates of cardiovascular disease (CVD) and related behavioral risk factors (Lee et al., 2013). Black Americans have been understudied in genome-wide association studies of diabetes and related traits. Klimentidis et al. (2012) reported an association between blood pressure and ancestry-informative markers near a marker identified by a genome-wide association study of ethnic and racial factors of systolic and diastolic blood pressure. They reported differences in risk factors for elevated blood pressure among ethnic/racial groups. Further, they emphasized the importance of including social and behavioral measures to fully explain the genetic/environmental etiology of disparities in blood pressure.

Inherited Variations Within Human Populations

Studying geographic subgroups is another way to understand race, ethnicity, and socially constructed variables. Luca and colleagues (2008) studied 12 population samples included in our study of NAT2 variation; these populations cover a geographic area extending from Africa north of the equator to south and east Europe and northeast Asia to the Beringian coast. The extremes of the geographic range include three African populations (Dendi from Nigeria and the Amhara and Oromo from Ethiopia) and a Siberian population from the Chukotka peninsula.

According to Weinshilboum and Wang (2004), a majority of inherited variations in drug response (pharmacogenetic traits) have involved drug metabolism. For example, one trait, which was recognized one-half century ago, is an inherited variation in N-acetylation, now known to be due to polymorphisms in the N-acetyltransferase-2 (NAT2) gene (Timbrell, Harland, & Facchini, 1980). Genetic variation in NAT2 is responsible for phenotypic variation in the pharmacokinetics and, therefore, the effects of drugs as different as hydralazine for hypertension and procainamide for dysrhythmia (Weinshilboum & Wang, 2004).

Furthermore, Irvin et al. (2011) examined the joint association of single nucleotide polymorphisms (SNPs) and copy number variants (CNVs) with fasting insulin and an index of insulin resistance (HOMA-IR) in the HyperGEN study, a family-based study with proband ascertainment for hypertension.

> **NOTE**
>
> *Proband* is a term used in medical genetics and other medical fields to identify a particular person being studied or treated. When whole families are studied for patterns of inheritance of genetic disorders, the proband is the first affected family member being treated.

These are just a few of the recent scientific reports on the evolving body of evidence that links complex genetic, environmental, and "social constructed" traits (including race and ethnicity) with variation in pharmacokinetics. The pace of discovery is overtaking (and will likely accelerate) the pace of nursing education and student learning.

Limited Funding for Nursing Research

The National Institutes of Health (NIH) Roadmap places a high priority on discovery and understanding of complex biological systems and the need to assemble teams of scientists with different and complementary perspectives and expertise. This may be interpreted to include nurse scientists who endeavor to study patient outcomes with respect to pharmacogenomics developments. There are limited funding opportunities available to systematically study creative approaches to presenting and translating this complex and dynamic body of knowledge to practicing nurses.

Is Nursing Ready?

Looking to the future and given the great promise of pharmacogenomics, one might predict a significant increase in the use of genetic testing prior to pharmacotherapy. Looking to the past at the guarded integration of genetics and pharmacogenomics in nursing education and practice, one might predict a deficiency in the ability of healthcare professionals to appropriately translate the science and educate patients and families. The broad scope of the results of genetic testing in general will require that patients receive complex and detailed information before they consent to being tested. The standard of care for predictive testing dictates that patients receive an explanation of the relevance of findings and recommendations for promoting or restoring health.

Easily understood and well-constructed instructional materials incorporating pharmacogenomics will be essential to assist patients to make informed decisions. This information will need to be continually updated and modified for general instruction, as well as updated and personalized to the situational factors and clinical profiles of individual patients.

A nurse who oversees the process of patient education on pharmacogenomics will find this responsibility daunting. Whole genome sequences will need to be reviewed regularly by teams of professionals to incorporate new information about risk and efficacy, and then change treatment strategies based on these assessments. Given the rapidity of scientific discovery and the translation of discovery to patient care, even advanced practice nurses will struggle to keep pace.

Looking ahead, there may be an insufficient number of genetic counselors to whom patients may be referred for additional information, and physicians will be coping with a growing cohort of patients for whom pharmacogenomics will be the standard of care (Ormond et al., 2010). Nurses may be required to step into an updated role and provide, at minimum, basic genetic/genomic information at the bedside. Working within the boundaries of the contemporary system of nursing education, patient workloads, and other professional expectations, attaining the ideal of best-practice patient education and follow-up seems, at this junction, perhaps impossible. Even with the intention to integrate genetics into the curriculum, faculty will struggle to keep pace with discovery.

Without assuring that nursing faculty embrace the relevance of advances in pharmacogenomics to patient care, contemporary nursing education will be producing graduates who will not be sufficiently prepared to take a significant role in bench-to-bedside translation.

Proposition: Personal Relevance Leads to Changes in Professional Practice

One way to counter this trend or prevent this portent is to systematically identify and study creative approaches to integrating this complex and dynamic body of knowledge with faculty preparation and student training. This is easier to state than achieve, but the instrumental link is "personal relevance."

Advocates of genetics and pharmacogenomics in nursing curricula imagine that these topics are relevant in and of themselves. This is error in judgment because of the great variation in personal experience and ability to comprehend the science. What is relevant to one person may be completely irrelevant to another, even when a teacher attempts to inculcate the set of ideas that should be embraced as valuable. Nursing curricula is replete with relevant information. That which is immediately and repeatedly used, in effect, shifts to the top. All the information provided to nursing students may be important and valuable but may not necessarily be relevant. Relevance implies having meaning or a specific connection to an individual. Information, albeit important, does not become relevant simply by being stated as such by an authority.

Thus, the challenge to nursing is to make pharmacogenomics more concrete and personal for each student and faculty and thereafter highlight its relevance beyond the personal context. Two questions, therefore, are before us:

- What may be the effect on learning, belief of relevance, and ability to translate to patient care if every nursing faculty and student is provided with their own genetic/genomic/pharmacogenomics testing and counseling?
- Are we ready?

QUESTIONS

Bench-to-bedside translation of pharmacogenomics would specifically include:

    a.   Three-generation family pedigree

    b.   Provision of genetic/genomic educational resources to patients

    c.   Assessment of the patient's personal genetic variants that affect drug response *

    d.   Assuring the patient provides informed consent

All the following are advantages of pharmacogenomics *except*:

    a.   Allows appropriate dose adjustment

    b.   Allows accurate monitoring of expected response

    c.   Informs alternative therapeutic selection before exposure to the drug

    d.   Prevents all occurrences of side and adverse events*

Describe the problem faced by nursing profession with regard to the integration of pharmacogenomics with patient care.

    All professions undergo rapid change and increasing specialization. With the rapid pace of discovery in genomics, nurses are having difficulty keeping pace with, learning, and translating new knowledge to practice in order to improve patient care. There is a wide range of educational preparation of the bedside nurse, from diploma school graduate to master's degree–prepared. There is also a wide range in the content and process of genetics instruction and the inclusion of pharmacogenomics in nursing curricula. This results in a population of practicing nurses who have varying degrees of interest in learning about, ability to apply, and belief in the relevance of pharmacogenomics to bedside nursing care.

Key Points

- Genetics core competencies can be adapted to add a focus on pharmacogenomics.

- Nursing faculty need specific preparation in genetics.

- Nursing faculty need further preparation on how to integrate pharmacogenomics with nursing curricula.

References

Becquemont, L. (2009). Pharmacogenomics of adverse drug reactions: Practical applications and perspectives. *Pharmacogenomics, 10*(6), 961–969.

Brantl, V. M., & Esslinger, P. N. (1964). Genetic implications for the nursing curriculum. *Nursing Forum, 1*(2), 90–100.

Burchard, E. G., Ziv, E., Coyle, N., Gomez, S. L., Tang, H., Karter, A. J., . . . Risch, N. (2003). The importance of race and ethnic background in biomedical research and clinical practice. *The New England Journal of Medicine, 348*(12), 1170–1175.

Burroughs, V. J., Maxey, R. W., & Levy, R. A. (2002). Racial and ethnic differences in response to medicines: Towards individualized pharmaceutical treatment. *Journal of the National Medical Association, 94*(10 Suppl), 1–26.

Collins, F. (1997). Preparing health professionals for the genetic revolution. *JAMA, 278*(15), 1285-1286.

Calzone, K., Cashion, A., Feetham, S. L., Jenkins, J., Prows, C. A., Williams, J., & Wung, S. F. (2010). Nurses transforming health care using genetics and genomics. *Nursing Outlook, 58*(1), 26–35.

Calzone, K., Jenkins, J., Prows, C. A., & Masney, A. (2011). Establishing the outcome indicators for the essential nursing competencies and curricul guidelines for genetics and genomics. *Journal of Professional Nursing, 27*(3), 179–191.

Calzone, K., Jerome-D'Emilia, B., Jenkins, J., Goldgar, C., Rackover, M., Jackson, J., . . . Feero, W. G. (2011). Establishment of the Genetic/Genomic Competency Center for Education. *Journal of Nursing Scholarship, 43*(4), 351–358.

Cooper, R. S., Kaufman, J. S., & Ward, R. (2003). Race and genomics. *The New England Journal of Medicine, 348*(12), 1166–1169.

Daack-Hirsch, S., Dieter, C., & Quinn Griffin, M. T. (2011). Integrating genomics into undergraduate nursing education. *Journal of Nursing Scholarship, 43*(3), 223–230. doi: 10.1111/j.1547-5069.2011.01400.x

Daack-Hirsch, S., Quinn Griffin, M. T., & Dieter, C. (2011). Integrating genomics into undergraduate nursing education. *Journal of Nursing Scholarship, 43*(3), 221–327.

Egan, B. M., Zhao, Y., & Axon, R. N. (2010). US trends in prevalence, awareness, treatment, and control of hypertension, 1988-2008. *JAMA, 303*(20), 2043–2050.

Genetics and Genomics Competency Center for Education (G2C2). Competency guidelines and curriculum map. Retrieved from http://www.g-2-c-2.org/start_search_map.php

Giarelli, E. & Reiff, M. (2012). Genomic literacy and competent practice: Call for research on genetics in nursing education. *Nursing Clinics of North America, 47*, 529–545. doi:10.1016/j.cnur.2012.07.006

Greco, K. (2008). Integrating ethical guidelines with scope and standards of genetics and genomics nursing practice. In R. B. Monsen (Ed.), *Genetics and ethics in health care: New questions in the age of genomic health*. Silver Springs, MD: American Nurses Association.

Greco, K. E., Tinley, S., & Seibert, D. (2011). *Essential genetic and genomic competencies for nurses with graduate degrees*. Silver Springs, MD: American Nurses Association and International Society of Nurses in Genetics. Available at http://www.nursingworld.org/MainMenuCategories/EthicsStandards/Genetics-1

Guttmacher, A. E., Porteous, M. E., & McInerney, J. D. (2007). Educating health-care professionals about genetics and genomics. *Nature Reviews Genetics, 8*(2), 151–157. doi: doi:10.1038/nrg2007

Hetteberg, C. G., & Prows, C. A. (2004). A checklist to assist in the integration of genetics into nursing curricula. *Nursing Outlook, 52*(2), 85–88.

Innocenti, F., & Ratain, M. J. (2004). "Irinogenetics" and UGT1A: From genotypes to haplotypes. *Clinical Pharmacology & Therapeutics, 75*(6), 495–500.

Irvin, M. R., Wineinger, N. E., Rice, T. K., Pajewski, N. M., Kabagambe, E. K., Gu, C., . . . Arnett, D. K. (2011). Genome-wide detection of allele specific copy number variation associated with insulin resistance in African Americans from the HyperGEN study. *PLoS ONE [Electronic Resource], 6*(8), e24052. Retrieved from http://www.plosone.org/article/info%3Adoi%2F10.1371%2Fjournal.pone.0024052

Jannetto, P. J., & Bratanow, N. C. (2009). Utilization of pharmacogenomics and therapeutic drug monitoring for opioid pain management. *Pharmacogenomics, 10*(7), 1157–1167.

Jenkins, J., Bednash, G., & Malone, B. (2011). Guest editorial: Bridging the gap between genomic discoveries and clinical care: nurse faculty are key. *Journal of Nursing Scholarship, 43*(1), 1–2.

Jenkins, J., Dimond, E., & Steinberg, S. (2001). Preparing for the future through genetics nursing education. *Journal of Nursing Scholarship, 33*(2), 191–195.

Jenkins, J., Grady, P., & Collins, F. S. (2005a). Nurses and the genomic revolution. *Journal of Nursing Scholarship, 37*(2), 98–101.

Jenkins, J., Grady, P., & Collins, F. S. (2005b). Nurses and the genomic revolutions. *Journal of Nursing Scholarship, 37*(2), 98–101.

Jenkins, J., & Lea, D. H. (2005). *Nursing care in the genomic era: A case-based approach*. Sudbury, MA: Jones & Bartlett.

Kegley, J. (2003). An ethical imperative: Genetics education for physicians and patients. *Med Law Review, 22*(2), 275–283.

Klimentidis, Y. C., Dulin-Keita, A., Casazza, K., Willig, A. L., Allison, D. B., & Fernandez, J. R. (2012). Genetic admixture, social-behavioural factors and body composition are associated with blood pressure differently by racial-ethnic group among children. *Journal of Human Hypertension, 26*(2), 98–107.

Lea, D. H., Feetham, S. L., & Monsen, R. B. (2001). Genomic-based health care in nursing: A bidirectional approach to bringing genetics into nursing's body of knowledge. *Journal of Professional Nursing, 18*(3), 120–129.

Lea, D. H., & Monsen, R. B. (2003). Preparing nurses for a 21st Century role in genomics-based health care. *Nursing Education Perspectives, 24*(2), 75–80.

Lea, D. H., Skirton, H., Read, C. Y., & Williams, J. (2011). Implications for educating the next generation of nurses on genetics and genomics in the 21st Century. *Journal of Nursing Scholarship, 43*(1), 3–12.

Lee, H., Kershaw, K. N., Hicken, M. T., Abdou, C. M., Williams, E. S., Rivera-O'Reilly, N., & Jackson, J. S. (2013). Cardiovascular disease among Black Americans: Comparisons between the U.S. Virgin Islands and the 50 U.S. states. *Public Health Reports, 128*(3), 170–178.

Lewis, J. A., Calzone, K., & Jenkins, J. (2006). Essential nursing competencies and curriculum guidelines for genetics and genomics. *Maternal Child Nursing, 31*(3), 146–153.

Lewis, R. (2012). *Human genetics: Concepts and applications* (10th ed.). New York, NY: McGraw Hill.

Luca, F., Bubba, L., Basile, M., Brdicka, R., Michalodimitrakis, E., Rickards, O., . . . Novelletto, A. (2008). Multiple advantageous amino acid variants in the *NAT2* gene in human populations. PLoS, (September 5). Retrieved from http://www.plosone.org/article/info%3Adoi%2F10.1371%2Fjournal.pone.0003136. doi: 10.1371/journal.pone.0003136

Marietta, A., Romero, K., & Malone, D. C. (2009). Warfarin interactions with substances listed in drug information compendia and in the FDA-approved label for warfarin sodium. *Clinical Pharmacology & Therapeutics, 86*(4), 425–429.

Marsh, S., & McLeon, H. L. (2004). Pharmacogenetics of irinotecan toxicity. *Pharmacogenomics, 5*(7), 835–843.

National Institutes of Health/National Human Genome Research Institute. (2014). Genetics/Genomics Competency Center for Education. Retrieved from http://www.g-2-c-2.org/

Nussbaum, R. L., McInnes, R. R., & Willard, H. F. (2007). The human genome: Gene structure and function (chapter 3, pp 25–39). In *Thompson & Thompson genetics in medicine*. Philadelphia: Elsevier.

Ormond, K. E., Wheeler, M. T., Hudgins, L., Klein, T. E., Butte, A. J., Altman, R. B., . . . Greely, H. T. (2010). Challenges in the clinical application of whole-genome sequencing. *The Lancet, 375*(9727), 1749–1751.

Osterberg, L., & Blaschke, T. (2005). Adherence to medication. *The New England Journal of Medicine, 353*(5), 487–497.

Snozek, C., Langman, L. J., & Dasgupta, A. (2012). Traditional therapeutic drug monitoring and pharmacogenomics: Are they complementary? In L.J. Langman, A. Dasgupta (Eds.) *Pharmacogenomics in Clinical Therapeutics* (pp15–25). Wiley-Blackwell. doi:10.1002/9781119959601.ch2

Stamer, U. M., Zhang, L., & Stuber, P. (2003). Personalized therapy in pain management: Where do we stand? *Pharmacogenomics, 11*(6), 843–864.

Timbrell, J. A., Harland, S. J., & Facchini, V. (1980). Polymorphic acetylation of hydralazine. *Clinical Pharmacology & Therapeutics, 28*(3), 350–355.

Weinshilboum, R., & Wang, L. (2004). Pharmacogenomics: Bench to bedside. *Nature Reviews Drug Discovery, 3*(9), 739–749.

Wilson, J. F., Weale, M. E., Smith, A. C., Gratrix, F., Fletcher, B., Thomas, M. G., . . . Goldstein, D. (2001). Population genetic structure of variable drug resonse. *Nature Genetics, 29*(3), 265–269.

Pharmacogenomics and Obstetric/ Prenatal Patients

Lynnette Howington, DNP, RNC, WHNP-BC, CNL

5

Pregnancy is a significant time of change. Change occurs physically and mentally to the expectant mother, the fetus undergoes change as he/she grows and develops daily, and there is change in the family dynamic when a child is expected. Healthcare providers strive to ensure each pregnancy is healthy, using current research and testing to help promote the same.

In doing so, providers need to recognize the significance of pharmacogenomics during pregnancy. The health of the mother during pregnancy can affect fetal development and pregnancy outcomes, and the expectant mother's health may in part be due to medication taken before or during pregnancy. A majority of women have taken at least one prescription or over-the-counter (OTC) medication before learning of their pregnancy (Iqbal, Audette, Petropoulos, Gibb, & Matthews, 2012; Ke, Rostami-Hodjegan, Zhao, & Unadkat, 2014). Providers need to know how medications may influence fetal development and the pharmacogenomic implications. When providers are aware of the effect of medications on the fetus, they can enter into a partnership with the expectant mother to discuss pregnancy concerns.

OBJECTIVES

- Understand the periods of fetal development and vulnerabilities.
- Discuss the FDA drug classification system for medications during pregnancy and the future of this classification system.
- Understand the risk to the fetus related to certain medications and substances taken during pregnancy.
- Discuss future directions in pharmacogenomic research as related to pregnancy and the fetus.

This chapter discusses some of the common medications and substances that need providers' attention during pregnancy and will highlight potential relationships between pregnancy and pharmacogenomics.

Fetal Development

When women actively plan their pregnancies, preconception counseling includes advising the woman to avoid using all over-the-counter medications, herbal remedies, illicit drugs, alcohol, and nicotine. Though some over-the-counter medications such as cold remedies and antacids are permitted during pregnancy, it is preferred that women discuss all medications with their provider before self-medicating when seeking pregnancy (Perry, 2012). During the preconception period, women on prescription medications should confer with their physician as to the safety of the medication for the developing fetus. Abrupt cessation of prescription medications can have untoward side effects, and this practice should be avoided (Patil, Kuller, & Rhee, 2011). However, women do not usually discover that a pregnancy exists until after a missed menstrual period. By the time the pregnancy is confirmed, the embryonic period is well underway, and major organ systems are already developing. The first 8 weeks of the gestational period are considered the most vulnerable to the influence of medications and teratogens, and the result can manifest in the form of fetal structural anomalies, spontaneous abortion of the fetus, or later behavioral or developmental delays during childhood. This section will further describe early fetal development, ways the maternal system and placenta protect the fetus, and drug classifications in pregnancy.

Early Fetal Development

The 40-week gestational period is divided into three periods: the preimplantation period, the embryonic period, and the fetal period.

- **Preimplantation period:** The time from fertilization to implantation in the uterine wall, considered a 2-week period.
- **Embryonic period:** Considered the time from week 3 to week 8. This period sees rapid organ development and is thus a time of extreme fetal vulnerability (Blumenfeld, Reynolds-May, Altman, & El-Sayed, 2010; Perry, 2012). During the embryonic period, the risk for teratogenic effects from medications is the

highest. Exposure to/intake of medications, viruses, cigarette smoking, and illicit substances during this time can cause fetal anomalies to the developing organ systems.

- **Fetal period:** Covers week 9 until the completion of pregnancy. This time sees organ maturation, weight gain, and body growth. During this period, the fetus is less vulnerable to teratogens, except for those that may affect the central nervous system, such as excessive alcohol use (Perry, 2012).

Table 5.1 shows important milestones of development during the early weeks of pregnancy.

Table 5.1   Periods of Fetal Development

Gestational Age	Development
Preimplantation period, week 1–2	The time from fertilization until implantation is a time of minimal to no risk by teratogens to cellular development.
Embryonic period, week 3–8	Cardiac system: weeks 3–9 Central nervous system: weeks 3–38 Limbs: weeks 4–9 Ears: weeks 4–30 Eyes: weeks 4–38 Lips: weeks 5–8 Palate: weeks 6–9 Teeth: weeks 6–38 External genitalia: weeks 7–38
Fetal period, week 9–remainder of gestation	Maturation of organs, rapid body growth, weight gain

Protection During the Embryonic and Fetal Period

Both the maternal system and the placenta offer protection from medication exposure to the fetus. Although some medications pass rapidly to the placenta and do affect the fetus, protective mechanisms are naturally in place. Providers need to recognize that these mechanisms may influence the amount of drug that reaches the fetus; accordingly, alterations in dosing or a change in drug may be indicated.

Maternal System

The first layer of protection from teratogens and drug exposure for the developing fetus is the maternal system. The liver metabolizes the medication or drug, and the process of biotransformation allows for elimination through urine or stool. These two features decrease the amount of medication that passes through the placenta to the fetus. Of consideration is the functionality of the liver and kidneys, medication dose, the pH of the medication, and the protein binding of the drug. Maternal genetic alterations of the CYP pathway—specifically, CYP2C9, CYP2C19, and CYP2D6—can alter metabolism of medications and therefore affect the concentration of medication that passes to the placenta. At this time, routine testing for alterations in the CYP pathway is not conducted (Blumenfeld et al., 2010; Devane et al., 2006; Perry, 2012).

Placenta

The next layer of protection from drug or substance exposure is the placenta (Blumenfeld et al., 2010; Devane et al., 2006; Iqbal et al., 2012; Perry, 2012). In order for a substance to pass to the fetal circulation, the substance must go through four layers: namely, the synctio- and cytotrophoblast layers, the intravillous stroma, and the fetal capillary wall (Blumenfeld et al., 2010; Perry, 2012). Other factors influencing medication affecting the fetus include dosage—and, therefore, concentration—of the medication in the maternal system; placental blood flow; and the degree in which the substance is metabolized before reaching the fetus. Substances with a low molecular mass, which include most antidepressants and antiepileptic medications, pass easily into the fetal circulation (Blumenfeld et al., 2010; Devane et al., 2006).

The placenta plays a role in drug metabolism through the expression of various enzymes. The CYP enzyme pathways are expressed in the placenta; therefore, alterations in the CYP pathway may affect the amount of medication reaching the fetus. Alterations specifically in alleles of the CYP2J2, CYP2C9, and CYP2D6 enzymes may affect drug metabolism in the placenta in that a drug may be rapidly or slowly metabolized. Other enzymes act as transport enzymes, affecting the amount of drug reaching the fetus. These transport enzymes are P-glycoprotein (ABCB1, P-gp), multidrug resistance proteins

(ABCC3, MRP2), and breast cancer resistance proteins (ABCG2, BCRP; Blumenfeld et al., 2010; Devane et al., 2006).

There is opportunity for more research on placental enzymes that affect drug metabolism and transport. Research may help providers adjust maternal drug dosing to ensure the least possible amount of medication is passed to the fetus. Because the genetic makeup of the placenta is determined by the fetus—not the mother—it is difficult to determine which genetic alleles related to drug metabolism and transport may exist for the fetus. This poses a challenge to providers when considering medication dosing. Another challenge to understanding fetal drug metabolism is recent research showing the fetal liver may express enzymes related to biotransformation that the neonate does not express (Blumenfeld et al., 2010; Devane et al., 2006). Therefore, research on neonates to determine possible enzymes expressed *in utero* would not yield the desired results.

Drug Classification System for Medications During Pregnancy

Medications are classified by the Food and Drug Administration (FDA) as to the potential of the medication to cause fetal anomalies. Although the designations of Category A and Category B are straightforward, categories C, D, and X are more complicated. In these cases, taking the medication should be a risk/benefit discussion with the healthcare team. The FDA categories for drug use in pregnancy are:

- **Category A:** Adequate and well-controlled studies have failed to demonstrate a risk to the fetus in the first trimester of pregnancy (with no evidence of risk in later trimesters).
- **Category B:** Animal reproduction studies have failed to demonstrate a risk to the fetus, and there are no adequate and well-controlled studies in pregnant women.
- **Category C:** Animal reproduction studies have shown an adverse effect on the fetus, and there are no adequate and well-controlled studies in humans; but potential benefits may warrant use of the drug in pregnant women despite potential risks.
- **Category D:** There is positive evidence of human fetal risk based on adverse reaction data from investigational or marketing experience or studies in humans, but potential benefits may warrant use of the drug in pregnant women despite potential risks.

- **Category X:** Studies in animals or humans have demonstrated fetal abnormalities, and/or there is positive evidence of human fetal risk based on adverse reaction data from investigational or marketing experience, and the risks involved in use of the drug in pregnant women clearly outweigh potential benefits.

A common assumption is that the categories are in ascending severity order, implying that an anomaly caused by a Class C medication would be less severe than an anomaly caused by a Class X medication. This assumption is false in that the same fetal anomaly can be caused by category C, D, and X. The categories are based upon the amount of research conducted regarding risk to the fetus or ancillary findings reported by care providers (Patil et al., 2011).

Because the current drug classification system is less specific than desired by providers, the FDA began looking for a more clear method with which to share drug information relevant to pregnancy and lactation. The process began in 2008; as of this writing, the FDA is completing the Pregnancy and Lactation Labeling Rule. Each medication will have a risk summary, data section, and clinical considerations (see Table 5.2). Advocates for this new labeling system believe that it will bring more comprehensive information to the providers when counseling patients regarding the usage of medications during the pregnancy and lactation periods (Howland, 2009; Patil et al., 2011).

Table 5.2   Overview of Pregnancy and Lactation Labeling Content

	General statement about background risk and medication
Pregnancy	
Fetal Risk Summary	Discusses the likelihood of developmental abnormalities and explains relevant risk based upon data
Clinical Considerations	Describes any known risk from drug exposure to mother and fetus
	Provides dosing information, reactions specific to pregnancy, and potential neonatal complications
Data	Presents human and animal data separately

Lactation	
Risk Summary	Characterizes the effects of drug on milk production and presence of drug in human milk
Clinical Considerations	Provides dose adjustments during lactation and strategies to minimize infant drug exposure
Data	Presents an overview of the data that are the basis for the information in Risk Summary and Clinical Considerations sections

Normal Physiological Changes During Pregnancy

Common physiological changes in pregnancy influence drug metabolism, clearance, and protein binding. These changes can affect therapeutic drug levels, and providers must be vigilant about therapeutic dosing, given that medication strengths or methods of dosing may need to be altered throughout the pregnancy. Discussing the effectiveness of medications at each prenatal visit is important. As shown in Table 5.3, physiological changes that can affect medication dosing include (but are not limited to) increased cardiac output, increased renal plasma blood flow, increased metabolism, and decreased intestinal motility (Campbell & Spigarelli, 2013; Devane et al., 2006; Frishman, Elkayam, & Aronow, 2012; Shea, Oberlander, & Rurak, 2012). Circulating serum albumin decreases, and plasma protein binding decreases (Briggs & Wan, 2006; Frishman et al., 2012; Ke et al., 2014). These factors affect the levels of bound and free drug concentration in the maternal system and can alter the effectiveness of prepregnancy doses.

Table 5.3	Changes in Pregnancy and the Effect on Drug Metabolism and Elimination
Variance	*Response*
Increased cardiac output	Drug metabolizes more rapidly
Decreasing serum albumin	Increase in unbound drug
Increased fluid volume	Less concentrated serum drug in maternal system
Decreased gastrointestinal motility	Drug stays longer in the gastrointestinal system, increasing metabolism and absorption
Increased metabolism	Drug metabolizes and clears more rapidly through the maternal system
Increased renal blood flow and glomerular filtration rate (GFR)	Drug clears more rapidly, which could lead to subtherapeutic effects

Conditions Requiring Medication

Ideally, women should not take any medications in the preconception period or during pregnancy, but some women have conditions that require daily medication, and the medication can affect the fetus in an untoward manner. Some common conditions include epilepsy, depression or other mood disorders, and adult onset acne. Medications for these conditions are necessary on a daily basis; thus, providers need to be able to recognize the effects that medications for the conditions may have on the developing fetus.

Epilepsy

Epilepsy is a common neurological condition in pregnant women (Campbell & Spigarelli, 2013). Although low, there are teratogenic risks to the fetus when mothers take antiepileptic drugs (AEDs), and clinicians must work to minimize these risks while at the same time strive for seizure control. For this reason, preconception counseling is highly recommended.

Recommended AEDs that can be taken during pregnancy are lamotrigine, carbamazepine, and phenytoin although the teratogenic effects can be as high as 10% (Blumfeld et al., 2010). Common teratogenic effects include hypospadias, spina bifida, orofacial clefts, malformations of the cardiovascular system, and craniofacial defects. Valproate should be avoided based upon the higher risk of fetal malformations. Newer medications have not been studied as rigorously as of this writing, and are therefore not recommended. Vitamin K and folic acid intake in the preconception period and first trimester has been shown to decrease the potential for teratogenic effects, and screening for neural tube defects during pregnancy is recommended. An amniocentesis to diagnose neural tube defects is not currently recommended for women taking AEDs (Campbell & Spigarelli, 2013).

Because of the expected and normal physiologic changes that occur during pregnancy, doses of AEDs may need to be adjusted to maintain seizure control, and serum therapeutic monitoring of drug levels is recommended. Some women with epilepsy have been shown to have a 17%–37% increase in seizure activity during pregnancy because changes (such as increased maternal metabolism) may lead to lower serum concentrations of AEDs in the maternal system. After delivery, dosing can return to pre-pregnancy levels, and breastfeeding is encouraged as long as the infant does not show signs of sedation (Campbell & Spigarelli, 2013).

Of interest, there is an increased risk for life-threatening dermatologic reactions for patients taking carbamazepine and phenytoin that have the human leukocyte antigen, major histocompatibility complex, class I, B (HLA_B*1502) genotype. The presence of this allele can lead to development of Stevens-Johnson syndrome or toxic epidermal necrolysis (TEN). Stevens-Johnson syndrome is characterized by extensive rash and blisters covering portions of the body, and TEN is characterized by blistering and peeling skin over large amounts of the body, which puts patients at risk for severe infection. Both conditions are treatable but severe. The FDA recommends genetic testing for the presence of this allele for those pregnant women needing to switch to carbamazepine or phenytoin during pregnancy (Campbell & Spigarelli, 2013).

Depression

In North America, as many as 20% of the female population of childbearing age takes medication for mood disorders, such as depression (Devane et al., 2006; Iqbal et al., 2012; Shea et al., 2012). Selective serotonin reuptake inhibitors (SSRIs) are commonly used to treat major and minor depression before, during, and after pregnancy. In most cases, women can continue taking SSRIs during pregnancy with careful evaluation for therapeutic effects of the medication.

Some women feel the need to stop taking antidepressants as soon as they learn of their pregnancy. However, women should not do so because withrdrawal symptoms may include nausea, anxiety, insomnia, and dizziness (Fleschler & Peskin, 2008). Instead, expectant mothers should consult with their care provider to discuss proper medication and any necessary alteration in dosing. Although many of the common SSRIs may be safely taken during pregnancy, studies show neonatal withdrawal symptoms and increased incidence of congenital malformations in women who took paroxetine (Paxil) during pregnancy (Cuzzell, 2006; Fleschler & Peskin, 2008; Patil et al., 2011). Paroxetine is not recommended for use during pregnancy but is compatible during breastfeeding (Patil et al., 2011).

Because of the normal physiological changes in pregnancy, doses of SSRIs in pregnancy may need to be altered (Patil et al., 2011). The peak plasma concentration for SSRIs is between 2 and 8 hours, and they are metabolized in the liver through the CYP pathways (Fleschler & Peskin, 2008). The most common enzymes in the CYP pathway for metabolizing SSRIs are 1A2, 2C9, 2C19, 2D6, and 3A4 (Devane et al., 2006; Patil et al., 2011; Shea et al., 2012). Variants in these pathways affect drug metabolism, which influences the amount of maternal drug concentration and may lead to higher levels of medication transmitted to the fetus. Typically, genetic testing for variance in the CYP enzymes is not conducted before initiating therapy or when adjusting doses; therefore, medication effectiveness should be discussed during prenatal visits (Shea et al., 2012).

Common medications used in pregnancy, such as antifungals, steroids, and medications for heartburn, may impact the effectiveness of SSRIs because they are metabolized by the same CYP enzymes. Nurses should inquire as to all medications, both prescription and OTC, at each prenatal appointment (Shea et al., 2012).

SSRIs cross the placenta easily (Fleschler & Peskin, 2008; Iqbal et al., 2012), and there is a possible correlation between SSRI use in the third trimester and adverse neonatal effects attributable to neonatal withdrawal after delivery. Studies indicate effects to the infant can be seen shortly after birth and may include respiratory distress, low birth weight, decreased tone, and feeding problems (Blumenfeld et al., 2010; Fleschler & Peskin, 2008; Iqbal et al., 2012; Patil et al., 2011). One suggestion to avoid neonatal discontinuation symptoms is to decrease the medication dose slowly late in the third trimester if the pregnant woman can tolerate the lower dose (Patil et al., 2011).

What about SNRIs?

Serotonin and norepinephrine reuptake inhibitors (SNRIs) are antidepressants that work by inhibiting reuptake of serotonin and norepinephrine. Examples of SNRIs are venlafaxine (Effexor) and duloxetine (Cymbalta). This class of medications has similar considerations to the medications in the SSRI class when considering changes brought about during the prenatal period. Dose adjustment may be required based upon normal physiological changes in pregnancy. Similar to medications in the SSRI class, third trimester dosing should be evaluated for the possibility of neonatal withdrawal symptoms, and breastfeeding is not contraindicated (Patil et al., 2011).

Acne

Isotretinoin (Accutane) is a commonly used medication for severe acne. This medication is a Category X medication because it can cause congenital defects to the fetus up to 35% of the time (Choi, Koren, & Nulman, 2013; Wolverton & Harper, 2013). Such anomalies include craniofacial, cardiac, and neurological deformities. Strategies are needed when a woman of childbearing age is taking this medication. Strategies include counseling regarding fetal anomaly risk, a negative pregnancy test result before beginning therapy, agreement to use two reliable forms of birth control, and pregnancy testing throughout therapy. In some instances, the female must sign waivers and informed consent documents stating her awareness of the risks should she become pregnant (Choi et al., 2013; Schonfeld, Amoura, & Kratochvil, 2009; Wolverton & Harper, 2013).

Labor and Antibiotics

Most antibiotics given to the laboring woman are compatible with the fetus and have no untoward effects on fetal development or infant behavior. Common antibiotics prescribed in labor include penicillins, clindamycin, and erythromycin (Briggs & Wan, 2006). Some antibiotics are contraindicated, however, during not only labor but also in pregnancy. The most commonly avoided antibiotics are tetracyclines, especially in the second and third trimesters, because they can have adverse effects on the development of fetal bones and teeth. Sulfonamides carry the potential to cause hemolytic anemia and jaundice in the newborn if given to a mother at the end of the third trimester. Nitrofurantoin, usually given for bladder infections, may cause hemolytic anemia to patients with glucose-6-phosphate dehydrogenase-deficiency (G6PD) if given late in the third trimester (Briggs & Wan, 2006).

Unsafe Behaviors

Unsafe behaviors in the form of ingesting substances that can lead to changes in fetal DNA should be avoided in pregnancy. Two popular behaviors, alcohol and nicotine intake, will be further explored. The effects of both behaviors on fetal development and alterations to gene expression have been well researched.

Drinking Alcohol

When a pregnant woman ingests alcohol, the fetus must rely on the maternal hepatic system to clear the alcohol from the mother's body. Genetic alterations in metabolism influence clearance rates, directly affecting the amount of alcohol reaching the fetus. Alcohol exposure during pregnancy has been shown to result in long-term effects, including structural malformations, cardiac anomalies, renal hypoplasia, mental delay, and altered facial features (Blumenfeld et al., 2010; Rodriguez, 2004). The combination of these effects is called fetal alcohol syndrome (FAS).

To date, it is unknown as to how much alcohol consumed during pregnancy will result in FAS. What is known is that alterations of enzymes that metabolize alcohol to acetaldehyde and acetaldehyde to acetic acid lead to increased clearance of alcohol. Persons with this enzyme alteration are associated with higher rates of alcohol abuse because they need a volume of alcohol to achieve the desired intoxicating effects (Blumenfeld et al., 2010). The genes CYP2E1, ADH1B, and ALDH2 play a role in encoding the enzymes that convert alcohol to acetaldehyde to acetic acid. Genetic testing for these alterations is not usually performed during pregnancy; therefore, due to the unknown amounts of alcohol that are necessary to result in FAS, it is recommended that pregnant women not consume any alcoholic beverages (Blumenfeld et al., 2010).

Smoking

As many as 15% of women in the United States smoke tobacco to some extent during pregnancy (Knopik, Maccani, Francazio, & McGeary, 2012). Nicotine use is associated with unfavorable neonatal outcomes, such as low birth weight, orofacial clefts, preterm birth, sudden infant death, and premature rupture of membranes (Blumenfeld et al. 2010; Knopik et al., 2012,; Shi et al., 2007). Nicotine is metabolized by the CYP2A6 pathway in approximately 80% of the population. Alleles of this pathway yield persons who have poor, slow, moderate, or increased enzyme activity and therefore different rates of nicotine clearance (Blumenfeld et al., 2010). Nicotine readily passes to the fetus through the placenta, and concentrations of nicotine in the fetus are higher than that of the mother (Shi et al., 2007).

Some studies have suggested that maternal smoking during pregnancy can be associated with an increased risk of behavioral alterations during childhood. There are risks of conduct disorders, antisocial behavior, and attention deficit hyperactivity disorder (ADHD; Knopik et al., 2012; Langley, Heron, Smith, & Thapar, 2012; McGrath et al., 2012). The genetics of these associations, however, is unclear (Langley et al., 2012). Although certain MAOA genotypes are associated with antisocial behavior, smoking is not thought to alter the fetus' MAOA genotype (McGrath et al., 2012). And although risks for behavioral alterations in childhood are low, care providers should discuss the risks of nicotine exposure during pregnancy with expectant mothers at each prenatal visit.

Genetic Counseling

For some couples, preconception genetic counseling or counseling during pregnancy is appropriate. Counseling during both periods allows a review of maternal and paternal health, heritage, and age, as well as any medications taken during the preconception or prenatal periods. Sessions provide an opportunity to discuss the status of current or potential pregnancies and the appropriateness of chromosomal analysis and testing.

Family and Individual Health History

Nurses have the responsibility while conducting a health history to be aware of possible red flags that may constitute a referral to a genetics specialist. Nurses need to discuss the possibility of suggesting such a referral when the expectant male or female have any of the following conditions in their personal or family history (Beery & Workman, 2012):

- Cystic fibrosis
- Sickle cell disease
- Tay-Sachs disease
- Thalassemias
- Developmental delay
- Congenital heart disease
- Chromosomal abnormalities
- Hemoglobinopathies
- Multiple spontaneous abortions

A person's heritage can increase the likelihood of genetic conditions. The nurse should ask the couple whether they identify strongly with a particular heritage. This heritage should be noted, and genetic conditions seen frequently in specific populations should be discussed. The following ethnicities have increased likelihood for certain genetic conditions (Beery & Workman, 2012):

- Amish: Hemophilia B
- Ashkenazim: Tay-Sachs disease, Gaucher disease, Factor XI deficiency
- African: Sickle cell disease, G6PD deficiency, beta thalassemia, lactase deficiency
- Chinese: G6PD deficiency, lactase deficiency
- Caucasian/English: Cystic fibrosis
- Irish: Phenylketonuria, neural tube defects
- Navajo Indians: Ear anomalies
- Polish: Phenylketonuria
- Scottish: Phenylketonuria, cystic fibrosis

The nurse should remain mindful of the couple's age as well as family history. A significant increase in the likelihood of a mother having a child with chromosomal abnormalities occurs after age 35. The most studied impact of maternal age on offspring is Down syndrome (DS). The rate of DS occurring in a woman younger than age 30 is approximately 1:900; after age 35, that risk increases to 1:385. At age 45, the risk rises to 1:30 (Beery & Workman, 2012; Van Riper, 2012).

Chromosomal Analysis and Testing for Inherited Conditions

Preconception genetic testing of parents helps couples know the likelihood that their offspring will inherit or carry a genetically linked condition. Knowledge of preconception test results can be used to help couples plan their families.

For example, couples with a family history of an inherited genetic condition, cystic fibrosis, may desire to have genetic testing to see if they are carriers of the condition. Results of genetic testing allow parents to make decisions about childbearing and offer care providers the opportunity to provide support and education before pregnancy occurs (Beery & Workman, 2012).

Pregnancy testing is available to expectant parents that can confirm the presence or absence of chromosomal abnormalities. Amniocentesis and chorionic villi sampling are examples of this type of test. These tests result in a detailed analysis of the fetal chromosomal makeup and can diagnose chromosomal abnormalities as early as 10 weeks (Beery & Workman, 2012).

Future Directions

Opportunities exist for pharmacogenomic advances in the future for pregnant women and their fetuses. As genetic tests for alterations in the CYP enzymes become more commonplace, clinicians will have the ability to choose the correct dosage of a medication based upon the speed with which the mother metabolizes medications. As scientists learn more about the effect of the placenta on drug metabolism, in addition to the maternal ability to metabolize medications, clinicians will be able to ensure therapeutic effects to the expectant mother without fearing toxicity to the fetus.

The advancing field of *epigenetics,* the study of changes in gene expression unrelated to a change in gene sequencing, offers clinicians the ability to counsel expectant parents in ways they have not been able to in the past. While scientists continue to learn the cumulative effect of how stress, diet, environment, and medications impact human DNA expression, more can be learned about the likelihood of disease in both children and adults.

By discovering why gene expression is "turned on" or "turned off," clinicians can further encourage positive habits and discourage negative ones, such as alcohol and nicotine intake during pregnancy. Scientists are exploring the "two hit"—or, in some circles, the "three hit"—theory, which avers a predisposition of the fetus based upon its uterine environment for a particular illness of a class of illnesses as gene regulation is altered during gestation. After delivery, usually in childhood, a trigger—such as illness or elements in the environment—then causes the condition to manifest (Daskalakis, Bagot, Parker, Vinkers, & Kloet, 2013; Lillycrop, 2011). More research is needed to discover the extent to which the fetal environment predisposes persons to develop heart disease, depression, obesity, asthma, and autoimmune disorders.

The opportunities in the future for more personalized medicine in pregnancy will help clinicians determine medication dosing and ensure a healthy environment during the gestational period.

Summary

Many factors during the pre-pregnancy and prenatal states—personal history, family history of the parental dyad, medications, and behaviors—all affect the genomics of the fetus. Many medications have been found to affect the fetus during development. Nurses must be aware of such medications and encourage the patient to discuss alternatives and/or the risks and benefits of continuing with a specific medication during pregnancy with their healthcare team. Nurses must have the knowledge regarding reasons for genetic re-ferral and offer guidance to patients who may benefit from genetics-focused care during pregnancy.

Questions

During the fetal period, which medication can affect tooth development, and is therefore contraindicated?

a. Penicillins

b. Tetracyclines *

c. Metronidazole

d. Clindamycin

When discussing the use of antiseizure medications in pregnancy, the nurse knows that:

a. The risk of seizures decreases during pregnancy, and dosages may need to be reduced.

b. The risk of fetal malformations is higher when the medication dose is high.

c. Serum levels of medication should be checked throughout pregnancy for therapeutic dosing. *

d. Breastfeeding will be discouraged as the medication passes to the breast milk.

References

Beery, T. A., & Workman, M. L. (2012). Genetics and genomics in nursing and health care. Philadelphia, PA: F. A. Davis Company.

Blumenfeld, Y. J., Reynolds-May, M. F., Altman, R. B., & El-Sayed, Y. Y. (2010). Maternal-fetal and neonatal pharmacogenomics: a review of current literature. *Journal of Perinatology, 30*(9), 571–579. doi:10.1038/jp.2009.183

Briggs, G. G., & Wan, S. R. (2006). Drug therapy during labor and delivery, part 1. *American Journal of Health-System Pharmacy, 63*(11), 1038–1045. doi:10.2146/ajhp050265.p1

Campbell, S. C., & Spigarelli, M. G. (2013). Pharmacology and pharmacogenomics of neurological medications used in pregnancy. *Clinical Obstetrics and Gynecology, 56*(2), 305–316.

Choi, J. S., Koren, G., & Nulman, I. (2013). Pregnancy and isotretinoin therapy. *Canadian Medical Association Journal, 185*(5), 411–413. doi:10.1503/cmaj.120729

Cuzzell, J. Z. (2006). Paroxetine may increase risk for congenital malformations. *Dermatology Nursing 18*(1), 68.

Daskalakis, M. P., Bagot, R. C., Parker, K. J., Vinkers, C. H., & de Kloet, E. R. (2013). The three-hit concept of vulnerability and resilience: toward understanding adaptation to early-life adversity outcome. *Psychoneuroendocrinology, 38*(9), 1858–1873. doi:10.1016/j.psyneuen.2013.06.008

Devane, C. L., Stowe, A. N., Donovan, J. L., Newport, D. J., Pennell, P. B., Ritchie, J. C., . . . Wang, J. (2006). Therapeutic drug monitoring of psychoactive drugs during pregnancy in the genomic era: challenges and opportunities. *Journal of Psychopharmacology, 20*(4 Suppl), 54–59. doi:10.1177/1359786806066054

Fleschler, R., & Peskin, M. F. (2008). Selective serotonin reuptake inhibitors (SSRIs) in pregnancy: a review. *Maternal Child Nursing, 33*(6), 355–361.

Frishman, W. H., Elkayam, U., & Aronow, W. S. (2012). Cardiovascular drugs in pregnancy. *Cardiology Clinics, 30*(3), 463–491. doi:10.1016/j.ccl.2012.04.007

Howland, R. H. (2009). Categorizing the safety of medications during pregnancy and lactation. *Journal of Psychosocial Nursing, 47*(4), 17–20.

Iqbal, M., Audette, M. C., Petropoulos, S., Gibb, W., & Matthews, S. G. (2012). Placental drug transporters and their role in fetal protection. *Placenta 33*(3), 137–142. doi:10.1016/j.placenta.2012.01.008

Ke, A. B., Rostami-Hodjegan, A., Zhao, P., & Unadkat, J. D. (2014). Pharmacometrics in pregnancy: an unmet need. *Annual Review of Pharmacology and Toxicology, 54*, 53–69. doi:10.1146/annurev-pharmtox-011613-140009

Knopik, V. S., Maccani, M. A., Francazio, S., & McGeary, J. E. (2012). The epigenetics of maternal cigarette smoking during pregnancy and effects on child development. *Development and Psychopathology 24*(4), 1377–1390. doi:10.1017/S0954579412000776

Langley, K., Heron, J., Smith, G. D., & Thapar, A. (2012). Maternal and paternal smoking during pregnancy and risk of ADHD symptoms in offspring: testing for intrauterine effects. *American Journal of Epidemiology, 176*(3), 261–268. doi: 10.1093/aje/kwr510

Lillycrop, K. A. (2011). Effect of maternal diet on the epigenome: implications for human metabolic disease. *Proceedings of the Nutrition Society, 70*(1), 64–72. doi: 10.1017/S0029665110004027

McGrath, L. M., Mustanski, B., Metzger, A., Pine D. S., Kistner-Griffin, E., Cook, E., & Wakschlag, L. S. (2012). A latent modeling approach to genotype-phenotype relationships: maternal problem behaviors, clusters, prenatal smoking, and MAOA genotype. *Archives of Women's Mental Health, 15*(4), 269–282. doi:10.1007/s00737-012-0286-y

Patil, A. S., Kuller, J. A., & Rhee, E. H. (2011). Antidepressants in pregnancy: A review of commonly prescribed medications. *Obstetrical and Gynecological Survey, 66*(12), 777-787.

Perry, S. E. (2012). Conception and fetal development. In D. L. Lowdermilk, S. E. Perry, K. Cashion, & K. R. Alden (Eds.), *Maternity & Women's Health Care*, 10th ed.(pp.270-288). St. Louis, MO: Mosby.

Rodriguez, M. M. (2004). Developmental renal pathology: its past, present, and future. *Fetal and Pediatric Pathology, 23*(4), 211–229.

Schonfeld, T. L., Amoura, N. J., & Kratochvil, C. J. (2009). iPledge allegiance to the pill: evaluation of year 1 of a birth defect prevention and monitoring system. *Journal of Law and Medical Ethics, 37*(1): 104–17.

Shea, A. K., Oberlander, T. F., & Rurak, D. (2012). Fetal serotonin reuptake inhibitor antidepressant exposure: maternal and fetal factors. *The Canadian Journal of Psychiatry, 57*(9), 523–529.

Shi, M., Christensen, K., Weinberg, C. R., Romitti, P., Bathum, L., Lozada, A., . . . Murray, J. C. (2007). Orofacial cleft risk is increased with maternal smoking and specific detoxification-gene variants. *The American Journal of Human Genetics, 80*(1), 76–90.

Van Riper, M. (2012). Clinical Genetics. In D. L. Lowdermilk, S. E. Perry, K. Cashion, & Alden, K. R. (Eds.), *Maternity & Women's Health Care*, 10th ed.(pp. 43–59). St. Louis, MO: Mosby.

Wolverton, S. E, & Harper, J. C. (2013). Important controversies associated with isotretinoin therapy for acne. *American Journal of Clinical Dermatology, 14*, 71–76. doi: 10.1007/s40257-013-0014-z

Pharmacogenomics in Pediatrics

Lisa Bashore, PhD, APRN, CPNP-PC, CPON
Heidi Trinkman, PharmD

6

All nurses—but pediatric nurses in particular—should have at least a basic understanding of the role that genetics, genomics, and drug safety and toxicity play (Howington, Riddlesperger, & Cheek, 2011). Pediatrics nurses who work in subspecialties—specifically oncology—should seek educational opportunities to enhance their knowledge in pharmacogenomics. The discoveries of the Human Genome Project have obligated scientists and clinicians alike to further investigate the role of genetics in medicine, and there has been an explosion of information and studies investigating as to the role of genetics in medication metabolism. The role of pharmacogenomics in medicine is growing because of the vast amount of information that scientists and clinicians are learning about the effects of medicines in both adults and children. The role of genetics and genomics in variations in pharmacokinetics can be explained in some way by how our DNA sequence responds to pharmacotherapy (Russo, Capasso, Paolucci, & Iolascon, 2011).

The focus of this chapter, however, is on the role of pharamacogenomics in the field of pediatric medicine. In the specialized case of pediatrics, evidence suggests that genetic variations may determine how children respond to medications (Stevens et al., 2013). Further, special consideration must be paid to adverse drug reactions (ADRs) in children.

OBJECTIVES

- Understand the challenges in examining pharmacogenomics in children.
- Discuss the development of adverse drug reactions in children.
- Review the various genetic aberrations present in a select pediatric population (cancers in children).
- List medications used in the treatment of children that are potentially impacted by pharmacogenomic variability.

Unfortunately, most of the aforementioned pharamacogenomic and pharmacokinetic information published and available has been on adults, with little light shed on pediatrics (Stevens et al., 2013). Having said that, pharmacogenomics testing (PGx) has been studied more widely in children in recent years to refine dosing strategies in order to identify genes that determine drug distribution, metabolism, absorption, excretion, and response to therapy in children (Moran, Thornburg, & Barfield, 2011). Studies have been conducted in children to specifically examine the role of genomics in drug metabolism, especially in the fields of pediatric oncology, pulmonology, endocrinology, neurology, rheumatology, and gastroenterology.

We lead off this chapter by discussing the difficulties of ADRs in children as well as the challenges in testing children in pharmacogenomic trials. Then, several of the drugs used for specific disease states in these pediatric specialty fields will be discussed.

> *Pharmacokinetics* is the interaction among drugs and the human body in relation to absorption, distribution, metabolism, and excretion.

Adverse Drug Reactions in Pediatrics

An important concept to consider in the study of pharmacogenomics in children is adverse drug reactions (ADRs), which ironically assist investigators and clinical practitioners in gaining more information on drug responses in children. Children are not merely "small adults," and accordingly, they react differently to medications and dosages. Historically, ADRs investigated in adults are not comparable with the etiology of ADRs in children, which has unfortunately led to significant toxicities in children (Rieder, 2012).

Further, we must acknowledge the ethical considerations of the inclusion of this young population in research (especially Phase 3 trials). Thus, limitations in the study of children in clinical trials as a vulnerable population have led to lack of understanding in ADRs in children (Castro-Pastrana & Carleton, 2011). However, these authors felt that using ethical reasons for not including children in such studies is an unfounded rationale, and one that may lead to greater ADRs in children. The Liverpool adverse drug reaction causality assessment tool was developed to assist in the identification and assessment of ADRs in children specifically and provides a stepwise approach to determine the presence of an ADR. See Figure 6.1.

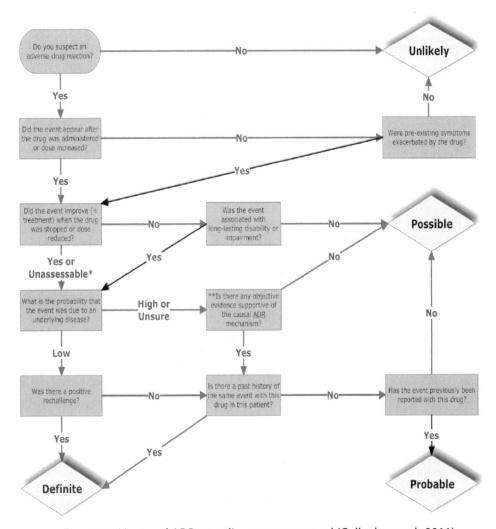

Figure 6.1 Liverpool ADR causality assessment tool (Gallagher et al., 2011).

Children may be more at risk for the development of ADRs due to many factors given the developmental changes occurring from infancy through adolescence. A vast number of children have experienced an ADR resulting in hospitalization or permanent injury—especially children diagnosed with leukemia (Rassekh, Ross, Carleton, & Hayden, 2013). The importance of reporting ADRs and understanding, documenting, and maintaining a database capturing ADRs is critical to understanding the patterns of their development (Carleton, 2010).

Combining what we have learned in the past from communication of ADRs and the current era of pharmacogenomics, using pharmacogenomics data in predicting the development of ADRs in children may prevent the occurrence of serious ADRs (Castro-Pastrana & Carleton, 2011). These same investigators have also made a very robust argument for the communication, documentation, and strict adherence to reporting and analysis of genetic markers for the development of ADRs in pediatrics.

Challenges in Pharmacogenomic Trials in Pediatrics

Many challenges exist in the study of pharmacogenomics in children: clinical trial investigations, lack of documented ADRs in pediatrics, and the developmental differences between children and adults. Documentation of ADRs in adults cannot be extrapolated to what may occur in children, especially young children. When considering pharmacogenomic research in pediatrics, other factors must be considered, such as obtaining consent, sample collections (which usually require invasive techniques), and possible reluctance on the behalf of both parents and the child (Freund & Clayton, 2003; Hawcutt, Thompson, Smyth, & Pirmohamed, 2013).

Despite these challenges, though, much has been learned from the investigation of drug therapy and safety through the use of pharmacokinetic studies using children. For example, studies investigating children with attention deficit hyperactivity disorder (ADHD) and acute lymphoblastic leukemia (ALL) specifically have contributed vastly to the current knowledge in pediatric pharmacogenomics (Hawcutt et al., 2013).

In 2002, the United States government and the Food and Drug Administration (FDA) created a method to increase the number of investigations to study drug therapy in children, and the Best Pharmaceuticals for Children Act of 2002 was enacted (Freund & Clayton, 2003). This act allowed the secretary of the U.S. Department of Health & Human Services (HHS; www.hhs.gov) to allocate monies from the National Institutes of Health (NIH) to direct funds to increase pharmaceutical studies in children. However, Moran et al. (2011) have reported that despite the potential benefits of pharmacogenomics testing in children, issues of reimbursement and the costs to healthcare for such testing remain present.

Genetics resources from NIH can be found at

http://ghr.nlm.nih.gov

Major challenges when investigating drug safety and toxicity in children are the developmental changes occurring throughout the early years and then changes in gene expression over time, especially in childhood. Because the tissues, organs, and cells in children are in different developmental stages throughout childhood, drug effectiveness may be associated with physiological maturation. As a result, pharmacogenomics studies may increase the understanding of this relationship (Joly, Sillon, Silverstein, Krajinovic, & Avard, 2008). Unfortunately, the feasibility of studying drug toxicity and safety in children over the course of their development is not possible (Freund & Clayton, 2003).

Differences in drug metabolism are a direct result of the contribution of genetic variations and ontogeny throughout the developmental stages in children. Many changes occur in children at the time of birth until and through adolescence, including rapid organ growth, and result in the variability in metabolism (Leeder, 2003). These differences account for much of the variation in pharmacokinetics, safety, and response to therapy.

> *Ontogeny* refers to the evolution of a species. In this case, it refers to the evolutionary history occurring during the developmental stages in children.

Developmental Aspects of Pharmacogenomics in Pediatrics (0–21 years)

This section discusses the developmental variations in children (0–21 years) that make studying pharmacogenomics in this population difficult.

In studies, many times the adolescent and young adult (13–21 years) population is not extracted and looked at separately as its own entity but is rather combined with children and evaluated as a whole. This makes separating out specific changes unique to adolescents and young adults very difficult to detect, and until more studies are performed looking at this unique subgroup of pediatrics, we won't be able to separate out the results

An individual's genotype does not change throughout his/her lifetime; however, the expression of that genetic information can change significantly from the neonatal period through adolescence (Hawcutt et al., 2013; Leeder, 2004). During this time period, organs and metabolic pathways mature alongside receptor systems and neuronal pathways being established (Neville, Becker, Goldman, & Kearns, 2011), creating a complex and layered picture when trying to evaluate interpatient variability with respect to response or toxicity from medications or environmental toxins. Ultimately, the hope is to be able to predict the response, dose needed, or risk of toxicity from a medication by using the patient's genetic information. Unfortunately, the paucity of data on children regarding drug dosing and disposition is further complicated by the inability to extrapolate pharmacogenomic findings from adult research due to the developmental differences in genetic expression.

Neonates (0–30 days) and Infants (1–24 months)

After the umbilical blood supply has been discontinued, the neonatal liver begins to take on many different biosynthetic and detoxification functions necessary for extrauterine adaptation. This new functionality includes aerobic metabolism, gluconeogenesis, coagulation factor synthesis, and bile production and transport (Leeder & Kearns, 2012). Microbial colonization also begins at birth with the composition being affected by mode of delivery, diet, hospitalization, and antibiotic therapy. The colonization, in conjunction with postnatal changes in hepatic function, can affect the ontogeny of drug biotransformation. Formula-fed infants acquire CYP1A2 activity more rapidly than do breast-fed infants (Leeder & Kearns, 2012), which makes predicting the pharmacodynamics and pharmacokinetics of drugs in this population very challenging.

Pediatric Pharmacogenetics in Action

Ward et al. (2010) conducted a study on the effect of CYP2C19 ontogeny on weight-normalized plasma clearance (CL/F) of orally administered pantoprazole. Postnatal age was positively correlated with CL/F in a cohort of neonates (N = 33) with ages ranging from 1 to 19 days. Interestingly, two neonates had a genotype for CYP2C19, considered predictive for poor metabolizers (PM). One neonate with the PM genotype, who was less than 4 days old, displayed a CL/F that was indistinguishable from the CL/F of four neonates with a genotype typically associated with an extensive-metabolizer phenotype. This demonstrates that ontogeny obscured the predicted clearance based on pharmacogenetic genotype (Ward et al. 2010).

After the first week of life, the fetal CYP3A7 rapidly declines as the CYP3A4/3A5 expression begins to increase dramatically, reaching 30% of adult levels by 1 month of age (Hawcutt et al., 2013). *In vitro* studies have shown that CYP2E1 expression surges within hours of birth, followed closely by the onset of CYP2D6 expression. CYP2C9 expression also begins to appear during the first week of life (Leeder, 2003). UGT has only 1% of adult activity level at birth but rapidly increases to adult levels by 14 weeks (Hawcutt et al., 2013). The lack of maturation in the glucuronidation pathway in neonates and exposure to the drug chloramphenicol is believed to be a major factor in the susceptibility of these babies to "gray baby syndrome."

Other systems, such as the protective efflux pumps, tend to mature a little slower. P glycoprotein (P-gp) expression in enterocytes increases rapidly within the first 3 to 6 months of life but doesn't reach full adult maturation levels until approximately 2 years of age (Neville et al., 2011). Enterocytes are the predominant cells in the small intestinal mucosa. They are tall, columnar cells and are responsible for the final digestion and absorption of nutrients, electrolytes, and water. P-gp expression in the blood-brain barrier also increases with postnatal age and demonstrates that these developmental patterns of expression may also be tissue-specific (Neville et al., 2011).

The last hepatic CYP to be acquired is CYP1A2, which has a significant delay in expression until 1 to 3 months of life (Leeder, 2003). Preliminary data from a longitudinal phenotyping study during the first year of life shows that with CYP2D6, the phenotype and genotype are in concordance by the second week of life as demonstrated by dextromethorphan O-demethylation activity. However, the ability to form N-demethylated metabolites—thought to be a function of CYP3A or CYP2B6 activity—is not only acquired during the first 2 to 4 months of life, but actually exceeds adult capacity at 1 year of age (Leeder, 2003).

> *P-glycoprotein* is a protein associated with tumor multidrug resistance. It acts as an energy-requiring efflux pump for many classes of natural products and chemotherapeutic drugs.

Effect of Pharmacogenomics in Specific Pediatric Disease States

In this next section, we attempt to gather and filter the sporadic pediatric pharmacogenomic findings as they pertain to medications commonly used in specific disease states seen in the pediatric population. The disease states with the most available data for consideration are pediatric acute leukemia, pediatric asthma, pediatric rheumatology, and ADHD.

Pediatric Malignancies

Developmental pharmacogenomic variability can have a profound impact on the efficacy and toxicity of medications used to treat pediatric diseases. One of the best examples of a disease state whose outcomes and toxicities are reflective of this variability is that of pediatric acute leukemias. Several of the chemotherapeutic agents that form the foundation of therapy for these children are impacted by pharmacogenomic variations in the pediatric patient population. Two well-defined examples of this include the abundantly studied genetic variation in children with respect to drug distribution, metabolism, and elimination of thiopurine methyltransferase (TPMT) and its effects on thiopurine metabolites 6-mercaptopurine (6-MP) and 6-thioguanine (6-TG; Pinto, Cohn, & Dolan, 2012). These two antimetabolites are prodrugs hepatically metabolized through multiple enzymes to their active moieties thioguanine nucleotides (TGN). TPMT is necessary for hematopoietic cells to inactivate these active metabolites (Pinto et al., 2012).

In 1980, Weinshilboum and Sladek were the first to characterize patients with absent erythrocyte TPMT activity. Subsequent studies showed that patients with erythrocyte-deficient TPMT were more prone to 6-MP related toxicities. Conversely, those patients with high erythrocyte concentrations of TPMT had an increased risk of relapse of their disease when treated with conventional dosing (Pinto et al., 2012). Although 24 variant alleles have been identified to date for the TPMT expression variability, only three—TPMT*2 (Ala80Pro), TPMT*3A (Ala154Thr and Tyr240Cys), and TPMT*3C (Tyr240Cys)—account for more than 95% of either low or intermediate TPMT enzyme activity (Rassekh et al., 2013; Russo, Capasso, Paolucci, & Iolascon, 2011). Roughly, 3% to 14% of patients are heterozygous for these variant alleles and are at intermediate risk of drug-related toxicity, which may indicate a dose reduction of 35% to 50% (Pinto et al., 2012; Russo et al., 2011). Patients who are homozygous for these variants are at high risk of severe toxicity and may require a >90% dose reduction (Russo et al., 2011).

Roughly 1 in 300 patients are homozygous for the nonfunctioning TPMT alleles based on population genomics (Leeder, Lantos, & Spielberg, 2010). Low TPMT activity is not only related to drug toxicity but also potentially to the risk of developing secondary malignancies, as seen in the St. Jude Children's Research Hospital ALL trial and replicated in the Nordic Society of Pediatric Hematology and Oncology trial (Rassekh et al., 2013). In the St. Jude Total XII trial, patients received cranial radiation concurrently with 6-MP.

The 8-year cumulative incidence of secondary brain tumors was found to be 42.9% in patients with low TPMT activity compared with only 4.7% in those with normal TPMT activity (Rassekh et al., 2013).

Although TPMT testing is not routine, it is incorporated into the evaluation of unexpected toxicity, with doses adjusted accordingly. Increasing recommendations by the U.S. FDA and international groups to incorporate genetic testing for these pharmacogenetic variables make TPMT testing highly likely to become integrated into frontline therapy.

Methotrexate

Methotrexate is an important chemotherapeutic agent used to treat several childhood malignancies (leukemia, brain tumors, and osteosarcomas) as well as some nonmalignant conditions, such as rheumatoid arthritis and lupus nephritis (Rassekh et al., 2013). Methylenetetrahydrofolate reductase (MTHFR) is an essential enzyme in the folate/methotrexate metabolic pathway. It has been found to have polymorphic variants, which yield proteins with a lessened activity level than the wild type. The variant of MTHFR (677C>; Ala222Val) encodes for a protein whose activity level is reduced to 30% of normal in approximately 10% of Caucasians. This variant has been associated with a higher incidence of toxicity (hepatotoxicity, neurotoxicity, mucositis) from methotrexate administration (Russo et al., 2011).

Another source of pharmacogenomic variability that has been studied in regard to methotrexate toxicity is the ABC superfamily of proteins (ABCB1, ABCC1-3, and ABCG2). These proteins are efflux pumps responsible for protectively pushing methotrexate out of cells. A recent study of 60 osteosarcoma patients demonstrated an association with methotrexate toxicity in patients with variants of MTHFR (A1958G; $p = 0.038$), ABCB1 (T3435C; $p = 0.027$), and ABCC2 (T3563A; $p = 0.028$; Windsor, Strauss, Kallis, Wood, & Whelan, 2012). A rather large study of 434 children with ALL demonstrated a correlation between toxicity, plasma concentration, and two highly linked SLCO1B1 variants (rs11045879 and rs4149081).

> A *superfamily* is a group of proteins having similarities, such as areas of structural homology, which are believed to descend from the same ancestral gene.

In addition to its potential contribution to risk of toxicity, the MTHFR single nucleotide polymorphisms (SNPs) may also affect efficacy of therapy. Aplenc et al. (2005) were the first to show the potential pharmacogenetic correlation of these SNPs with outcomes. The investigators evaluated 201 children with ALL from a single center and found that patients with the MTHFR T677A or the A1298C haplotype had a lower probability of Event Free Survival (EFS): hazard ratio (HR) 2.2, 95% confidence interval (CI) 0.9–5.6 (Aplenc et al., 2005). A Children's Oncology Group (COG; www.childrensoncologygroup.org) study, CCG Trial (1891) later supported this finding by looking at 520 patients with ALL who were genotyped for two common low-functioning polymorphisms (C677T and A1298G). Investigators reported that patients with the C677T SNP had a higher incidence of relapse (HR 1.82; $p = 0.008$) and was actually more predictive of relapse than the Day 8 bone marrow response (Krajinovic et al., 2004).

> *Haplotype* refers to the group of alleles of linked genes contributed by either parent.

Yang et al. (2009) completed studies in genome-wide association study (GWAS) investigating the SNPs most commonly associated with positive minimal residual disease (MRD) at end of induction and those associated with relapse in patients treated at St. Jude and from the Pediatric Oncology Group (POG) study #9906 for children with ALL. Yang and associates identified 102 SNPs associated with positive MRD at end of induction ($p < 0.0125$), and 21 of these were also associated with an increased risk of relapse (Yang et al., 2009; Yang et al., 2011). Several of these top SNPs were found in the IL15 gene, which is a cytokine that enhances proliferation and has been linked to steroid resistance. These SNPs were associated with a more aggressive clinical presentation of ALL at time of diagnosis as well as a higher incidence of central nervous system (CNS) relapse.

> POG was a predecessor to COG. POG combined with CCG (Children's Cancer Group) in the late 1990s to form the current international research consortium, COG. That being said, POG studies and CCG studies were continued to their completion as their original title and number under the COG umbrella. Each group had a slightly different approach to treating pediatric acute leukemias.

Vincristine

Vincristine is another chemotherapeutic agent widely used in the pediatric oncology population. Neuropathies are the most commonly seen toxicities associated with administering this drug. It has been demonstrated *in vitro* that vincristine is metabolized more efficiently by CYP3A5 than CYP3A4. Polymorphic expression of CYP3A5 may be a contributor to the pharmacokinetic variability and incidence of toxicities seen in pediatric oncology patients (Rassekh et al., 2013). A racial difference has been demonstrated between the incidence of vincristine-induced neurotoxicities between African American patients and Caucasians. This may be explained by the finding that more than 80% of African Americans carry at least one functional copy of the CYP3A5 allele, compared with only 10% to 20% of Caucasians (Rassekh et al,. 2013).

Researchers at Indiana University Simon Cancer Center evaluated the CYP3A5 genotypes for 107 pediatric patients treated for pre-B ALL (Egbelakin et al., 2011). They found that 82% of these patients were CYP3A5*3/*3 (CYP3A5 non-expressers) with only 18% CYP3A5 *1/*3 (CYP3A5 expressers). The incidence of neurotoxicity in the nonexpresser patients versus the expresser patients was found to be statistically significant ($p = 0.03$). Additionally, those patients found to be nonexpressers of CYP3A5 had significantly more vincristine doses reduced or omitted from therapy due to neurotoxicities than did the expressers ($p = 0.006$ and $p = 0.003$, respectively; Egbelakin et al., 2011).

> *Pre-B cells* are immature lymphoid cells that contain cytoplasmic IgM and develop into B lymphocytes.

Cisplatin

Cisplatin is a chemotherapeutic agent commonly used in the treatment of solid tumors in both children and adults. Cisplatin has considerable toxicities associated with administration, including emetogenicity, ototoxicity, peripheral neuropathies, and nephrotoxicity (Rassekh et al., 2013). There is considerable variability in cisplatin ADRs and evidence in adults that there may be racial differences in the incidence of cisplatin-induced toxicities. One study cites African-American patients as experiencing nephrotoxicity at a higher rate than Caucasian patients (47.6% vs. 8.3%; $p = 0.007$; Shord et al., 2006).

Unfortunately, there are no such studies yet in children. A recent study in adolescents with osteosarcoma studied eight SNPs in six genes. Only one variant (ERCC2) was found to be associated with a slightly better outcome. The largest pediatric study to date was published by the Canadian Pharmacogenomics Network for Drug Safety (CPNDS; www.

cpnds.ubc.ca), which identified two genes associated with cisplatin-induced ototoxicity: TPMT (OR 10.9-18.0) and COMT (OR 2.5-5.5). Patients who carried at least three or more risk alleles experienced a rapid decline in hearing, often as soon as first dose administration (Rassekh et al., 2013). Variants in one or both of these genes were able to explain nearly one half of all ototoxicity cases in the series.

Anthracyclines

Anthracyclines are a group of chemotherapeutic agents commonly used in both adults and children to treat a variety of solid and hematologic malignancies. One of the most worrisome toxicities with cumulative dosing is cardiotoxicity. More than 60% of pediatric cancer patients receive treatment regimens that include an anthracycline, and survivors of childhood cancers are 8 times more likely to die of heart disease and 15 times more likely to experience heart failure than their healthy contemporaries. The cardiotoxicity associated with anthracycline use can be immediate or long after the completion of therapy and is the second-most common cause of death among pediatric cancer survivors (Rassekh et al., 2013).

Despite certain patient-related risk factors being identified, there is still significant interpatient variability in the incidence of cardiotoxicity seen. The first pediatric retrospective study by The Childhood Cancer Survivor Study (CCSS; https://ccss.stjude.org/) looked at two specific polymorphisms (NQO1*2 and CBR3 V244M) in 30 cases of heart failure and found no statistically significant results (Blanco, Leisenring, & Gonzalez-Covarrusias, 2008). A report from Hungary reviewed 235 pediatric patients with ALL for nine polymorphisms in the ABCC1 gene. Semsei, Erdelyi, & Ungvari (2012) identified a variant (rs374527) that was potentially associated with lower-left ventricular ejection fraction (EF) seen after chemotherapy, which corresponded to the same gene identified in adult studies.

The largest pediatric trial to date was performed by the CPNDS investigating anthracycline-induced cardiotoxicity. Visscher, Ross, and Rassekh (2012) evaluated 344 patients, analyzing 2,977 genetic variants in 220 different drug biotransformation genes. A finding from this investigation was a highly significant association of cardiotoxicity with a coding variant within the SLC28A3 gene (rs7853758) with an odds ratio (OR) of 0.35 ($p = 1.8 \times 10^{-5}$). This study was then replicated in another study in 96 children from Amsterdam, in which the investigators also identified several additional variants, including SLC28A1, UGT1A6, ABCB1, ABCB4, and ABCC1 (Visscher et al., 2012).

> **Pediatric Cancer Genomic Project (St. Jude Children's Research Hospital and Washington University, St. Louis, MO)**
>
> http://www.pediatriccancergenomeproject.org/site/
>
> The Pediatric Cancer Genomic Project is a union between these two institutions to decode the genomes of 600 pediatric childhood cancer patients in an attempt to identify the genetic origins of pediatric malignancies. They will identify the genetic sequencing of both cancer cells and normal cells from each patient and compare the differences in the DNA to identify genetic mistakes that lead to cancer.

Pediatric Asthma

Asthma is the most common chronic disease among children. The treatment for acute exacerbations is most commonly agonists for the β2 adrenergic receptor (ADRB2). A common polymorphism in the coding region of the ADRB2 gene has had mixed results on the effectiveness of these medications when used in conjunction with inhaled corticosteroids in children (Russo et al., 2011). Two other therapeutic medications used in this patient population with known polymorphisms (CRHR1, LTC4, ALOX5) are the corticosteroids and the leukotriene modifiers.

Again, researchers have demonstrated contradictory results. A study conducted by Stockmann et al. (2013) evaluated the effect of nine different SNPs in the CYP3A4, CYP3A5, and CYP3A7 genes on inhaled corticosteroids and their effect on asthma control in pediatric patients. The investigators evaluated 734 children with asthma receiving an inhaled corticosteroid: fluticasone propionate. There was no correlation between SNPs in the CYP3A5 or CYP3A7 genes and asthma control. However, asthma control scores (scale of 0–15) were significantly improved in 20 children with the CYP3A4*22 allele by 2.1 points (95% CI, 0.5–3.8). The researchers' hypothesis is that CYP3A4*22 reduces metabolic enzyme activity, thereby increasing airway exposure to the steroid; however, the direct functional significance of this finding is unclear (Stockmann et al., 2013). More research including replication is warranted. Potentially this finding could lead to more pharmacogenetically tailored inhaled corticosteroid regimens in the future.

In addition to the potential role of polymorphisms on medications used to treat asthma in children, there could also be a potential for pharmacogenomics to play a role in the disease process itself, thus affecting the severity and response to treatment. One component of asthma is an Igor-mediated allergic response. IgE synthesis is mediated through IL-4 stimulation of B lymphocytes; therefore, IL-4 serves a disease-modifying role (Szefler, 2003). Two polymorphisms that could affect this synthesis altering the severity of disease are C589T (which increases IL-4 synthesis) and R576 (which increases the sensitivity of the IL-4 receptor). Failure to respond to treatment could potentially be due to excessive pathway activity or alternative pathways involved in the disease process (Szefler, 2003).

Pediatric Rheumatology

Methotrexate is a fundamental therapeutic agent in the treatment of both adults and children with rheumatoid arthritis (RA; Becker, 2012). As described earlier in this chapter, there is significant interpatient variability with regard to efficacy and toxicity. Pharmacogenomic investigations in adult patients with RA have identified several possible SNPs in amino imidazole carboxamide ribonucleotide transformylase (ATIC); reduced-folate carrier (SLC19A1); and inosine-triphosphate pyrophosphatase (ITPA), which through gene-gene interaction, may play a role in both toxicities and outcomes (Becker, 2012). These gene-gene interactions may contribute to differences in distribution of cellular biomarkers, such as methotrexate polyglutamate (MTXGlu), in patients with juvenile idiopathic arthritis (JIA). Individuals who carried an SNP combination of ATIC (rs4673990) and the adenosine receptor ADORA2a (rs3761422) were 18.5 times more likely to have low concentrations of the MTXGlu biomarker (95% CI 3.7–93.2; $p < 0.0001$).

Continued research needs to be conducted to determine the clinical significance of this finding. In 2011, the Childhood Arthritis Response to Medication Study (CHARMS) identified several possible candidate SNPs in ATIC and ITPA genes that seemed to indicate a poor response to methotrexate (Hinks, Moncrieffe, & Martin, 2011). The U.S. cohort used for validation did demonstrate a trend toward significance ($p = 0.07$) for the ATIC SNPs, but no potential proxies available for testing the ITPA SNPs.

Mycophenolate mofetil (MMF) has been gaining popularity as a treatment option in pediatric rheumatology. Mycophenolic acid (MPA) is the active metabolite of MMF that targets T and B lymphocytes through inhibition of inosine monophosphate dehydrogenase (IMPDH). MPA is further metabolized in several tissues by uridine diphosphate glucuronosyltransferases (UGT1A8, UGT1A9, and UGT2B7), which are known to have associated polymorphisms. There are still many areas of research into the genetic impact on variability of response in these patients with regard to TNF-α pathways and mitogen-activated protein kinase (MAPK) signaling networks. The findings of these studies are awaiting validation before further investigations are pursued and clinical impact can be evaluated (Becker, 2012).

Attention Deficit Hyperactivity Disorder

According to a survey of parents by the Centers for Disease Control and Prevention, approximately 6.4 million children ages 4 to 7 had been given a diagnosis of ADHD in 2011 (CDC, 2013). The prevalence of children ages 4 to 7 years taking medications for ADHD increased from 4.8% in 2007 to 6.1% in 2011 (CDC, 2011). A number of these children may not be receiving the full benefit from their medications (typically stimulants and/or antipsychotics) due to pharmacogenetic variations.

Hawcutt et al. (2013) alluded to the plethora of studies examining the pharmacogenomic implications in ADHD and other disease entities, but with varying interpretations. The need for ongoing pharmacogenomic studies in the medical management of children with ADHD is described in an update on the impact of known pharmacogenomic variations on the medications used in the treatment of this disease (Kieling, Genro, Hutz, & Rohde, 2010). These investigators examined more than 30 studies that evaluated the use of stimulant and psychotropic medications in children and adolescents with ADHD and the gene rearrangements and variants associated with their response. Unfortunately, there are disparate findings among the studies, thus making it difficult to establish guidelines for medication prescribing and administration.

The genetic aberrations reviewed included the dopamine transporter (DAT), and specifically the SLC6A3 (DAT1) gene, located on chromosome $5_p15.3$, which has been associated with methylphenidate response. Based on the number of allele copies 10/10, children were categorized as either poor or very good responders; unfortunately, studies tended to contrast each other lending to other factors to explain the findings (Kieling et al., 2010). The DRD4 gene is found on the $11_p15.5$ chromosome, specifically the 48-bp VNTR in exon 3 and reported to be associated with ADHD treatment response. Similar to the DAT1 gene, studies examining the DRD4 gene and response to methylphenidate are mixed.

The CYP isoenzymes CYP2D6 and CYP2C19 are responsible for the metabolism of many antidepressants and antipsychotics. CYP2D6 specifically metabolizes many of the psychotropic medications used in the treatment of ADHD.

Pediatric Pharmacogenetic Testing

A recent case report illustrates the value in pharmacogenetic testing in children to assure optimal therapeutic response to drug therapy for ADHD (Tan-Kam et al., 2013). A 6-year-old boy was originally prescribed methylphenidate 5mg tablets to be taken at 7 a.m. and then again at 12 p.m. He reportedly experienced markedly worsened disobedience, more impulsivity, poor appetite, and mischievous behaviors. After a thorough investigation, including an All-in-One PGx (CYP2D6, CYP2C19, and CYP2C9 were screened), the results indicated this young boy had a CYP2D6 *2/*10 genotype and was an intermediate metabolizer for this particular enzyme. This finding explained the adverse response to the medications he was given, including methylphenidate, haloperidol, and imipramine. His dose of methylphenidate was reduced to 2.5 mg each morning, and his behavior returned to normal.

The amount of new information being collected in the identification of genetic variations in children is increasing due to the lack of appropriate response to therapy despite proper dose administration of medications in the management of ADHD. Future studies are necessary to elucidate the varying responses to treatment for ADHD and to overcome the historical methodological issues from previous studies, including the lack of randomized control trials, definitions of even rare genotypes for ADHD diagnosis and treatment, and the lack of large databases in which to study this phenomenon. The new generation of large data sets will hopefully set the stage for more rigorous evaluation of ADHD treatment responses and advance the research and control over the manifestations of ADHD in all children.

Pharmacogenomics of Specific Medications Used in Pediatric Patients

As more and more research is being done in the area of pharmacogenomics and its impact on response to medications, it is important to keep in mind those medications used in pediatric patients as well as adults and determine the clinical significance of their findings. Table 6.1 is a compilation of medications utilized in the pediatric patient population, their pediatric pharmacogenomics findings, and associated SNPs.

Table 6.1 Medication-Related Polymorphisms		
Drug	*Findings*	*SNP*
Abacavir	Patients positive for this allele are at significant risk of hypersensitivity reactions. (Burchart & Green, 2012)	HLA-B*5701
Tacrolimus	Patients may need higher doses to attain therapeutic levels. (Manickaraj & Mital, 2012)	CYP3A5 expresser genotype
Oseltamivir	Use is associated with a higher incidence in neuropsychiatric adverse events possibly due to enhanced permeability of the blood-brain-barrier. (L'Huillier et al., 2011)	ABCB1 polymorphisms
Methylphenidate	Use is associated with positive response to methylphenidate for autism spectrum disorders. (McCracken, Badashova, & Posey 2014)	SLC6A4, SLC6A3, DRD1, DRD3, DRD4, COMT, ADRA2A
Deferasirox	Patients carrying two affected haplotypes were at increased risk of developing hepatotoxicity. (Lee et al. 2013)	MRP2 (−1774 del and/or −24T)

Future Directions

Investigators and the population have learned much from the identification of the Human Genome Project and the pharmacogenomics variations found in the pediatric population. However, there continues to be a dearth of information regarding the developmental differences in the pediatric population. Leeder (2004) reported that because of the dynamic processes of pharmacologic modulation of developing receptor systems, and networks resulting in response to drug therapies in children given drugs at a young age, the effects of the medications may not become apparent until later stages of the maturation process. Therefore, ongoing investigations in pharmacogenomics and pharmacogenetics need to include dimensions of a particular disease or process and their phenotypes that may change during development of the pediatric patient.

The U.S. FDA (2014) recently initiated a program—the Sentinel Initiative—to improve drug safety in all individuals, including children. This program allows for a prompt and swift approach in reporting drug toxicity and safety information to clinicians in practice to improve children's health through formal research initiatives in pharmacogenomics.

www.fda.gov/Safety/FDAsSentinelinitiative/ucm2007250.htm

Despite what we have learned in the field of pharmacogenomics in pediatrics, more continues to need to be done to advance the science and our knowledge in this field. Children do benefit from participating in clinical trials, and the research in pediatric hematology and oncology has revealed the value in understanding the mechanisms of action and the pharmacokinetics of the various chemo-toxic drugs used and their impact on outcomes (Aplenc et al., 2005; Davies et al., 2008; Visscher et al., 2012).

The discoveries made by the Human Genome Project and the implications that genetic testing has on the identification of various genetically powered diseases in children will further affect clinical practice and treatment. The ultimate goal is to improve health and survival either from genetic disease or prevention of ADRs in children. Wade, Tarini, and Wilfond (2013) reviewed the impact of growing up in the genomic era and surmised that the goal will be to capture data on whether the pediatric whole-genome sequencing (PWGS) influences health behaviors and health outcomes (survival). Furthermore, they suggested that clinicians, scientists, and policymakers need to be well prepared regarding the impact that using PWGS will have in guiding care and educating parents and children. What will the benefit be to families knowing their genetic risks for disease?

With the discoveries of the Human Genome Project, there are many opportunities for both the medical and nursing disciplines to take what has been learned from the laboratory to the bedside. Parents of children with serious health problems are seeking health information via the Internet and finding current medical information specific to their child's disease. This information often is representative of the newest drugs and other medical treatments, many of which have genomic undertones. It is vital that nurses at all levels understand the concept of pharmacogenomics to speak intelligently with their colleagues and to understand the mechanisms of the medications they administer to their patients.

Nursing researchers have many opportunities to contribute to the knowledge base of pharmacogenomics by collaborating with basic scientists to further their understanding of pharmacogenomics.

Questions

Why is it difficult to identify and understand the pharmacogenomic risk for ADRs in young children?

> Developmental changes occurring include the pharmacokinetics of drugs due to gene activity. The current research is limited in children and is primarily done in the adult population.

How do genetic polymorphisms in the TPMT gene affect patients being treated with leukemic malignancies?

> TPMT is necessary for hematopoietic cells to inactivate the active metabolites of 6-mercaptopurine and 6-thioguanine. Any variability in these enzymes can lead to excessive toxicities if underexpressed or a decrease in efficacy with ramifications on overall outcomes if overexpressed.

After delivery, microbial colonization begins and is affected by many factors. Name some of those factors.

> Delivery, diet, hospitalization, and antibiotic therapy

What gene activity develops faster in formula-fed babies? What are the results?

> Formula-fed infants acquire CYP1A2 activity more rapidly than breast-fed infants, which makes predicting the pharmacodynamics and pharmacokinetics of drugs in this population very challenging.

Key Points

- Pediatrics nurses working in various subspecialties of clinical pediatrics need to have a basic understanding of the potential impact of pharmacogenomics and pharmacogenetics of the drugs used to treat children of all ages.

- Developmental variations in neonates through early adolescence influence the variability in how they metabolize drugs and can result in serious ADRs.

- Challenges in overcoming developmental variability in pharmacokinetics, safety, and metabolism may warrant research difficult to perform in young children.

References

Aplenc., R., Thompson, J., Han, P., La, M., Zhao, H., Lange, B., . . . Rebbeck, T. (2005). Methylenetetrahydrofolate reductase polymorphisms and therapy response in pediatric acute lymphoblastic leukemia. *Cancer Research, 65*(6), 2482–2487.

Becker, M. (2012). Pharmacogenomics in pediatric rheumatology. *Current Opinions in Rheumatology, 24*(5), 541–547. doi:10.1097/BOR.0b013e3283556d13

Blanco, J., Leisenring, W., & Gonzalez-Covarrusias, V. (2008). Genetic polymorphisms in the carbonyl reductase 3 gene CBR3 and the NAD (P) H: quinone oxidoreductase 1 gene NQO1 in patients who developed anthracycline-related congestive heart failure after childhood cancer. *Cancer 112*(12), 2789–2795.

Burchart, G., & Green, D. (2012). The personalized medicine revolution: getting it right for children. *Pediatric Transplant, 16*(6), 530–532. doi:10.1111/j.1399-3046.2011.01638.x

Carleton, B. (2010). Demonstrating utility of pharmacogenetics in pediatric populations: Methodological considerations. *Clinical Pharmacology & Therapeutics, 88*(6), 757–759. doi: 10.10138.cipt.2010.242

Castro-Pastrana, L., & Carleton, B. (2011). Improving pediatric drug safety: Need for more efficient clinical translation of pharmacovigilance knowledge. *Journal of Population Therapeutic Clinical Pharmacology, 18*(1): e76–e88.

Centers for Disease Control and Prevention (CDC). (2013). Attention Deficit Hyperactivity Disorder. Retrieved from http://www.cdc.gov/ncbddd/adhd/data.html

Davies, S., Borowitz, M., Rosner, G., Ritz, K., Devidas, M., Winick, N., . . . Relling, M. (2008). Pharmacogenetics of minimal residual disease response in children with B-precursor acute lymphoblastic leukemia: A report from the Children's Oncology Group. *Blood, 111*(6), 2984–2890. doi:10.1182/blood-2007. 09.114082

Egbelakin, A., Ferguson, M., MacGill, E., Lehmann, A., Topletz, A., Quinney, S. K., . . . Renbarger, J. (2011). Increased risk of vincristine neurotoxicity associated with low CYP3A5 expression genotype in children with acute lymphoblastic leukemia. *Pediatric Blood & Cancer, 56*(3), 361–367. doi:10.1002/pbc.22845

Freund, C., & Clayton, E. (2003). Pharmacogenomics and children: Meeting the ethical challenge. *American Journal of Pharmacogenomics, 3*(6), 399–404.

Gallagher, R., Kirkham, J., Mason, J., Bird, K., Williamson, P., Nunn, A., . . . Pirmohamed, M. (2011). Development and inter-rater reliability of the Liverpool adverse drug reaction causality assessment tool. *PLoS ONE, 6*(12): e28096. doi:10.1371/journal.pone.0028096

Hawcutt, D., Thompson, B., Smyth, R., & Pirmohamed, M. (2013). Paediatric pharmacogenomics: An overview. *Archives of Diseases in Children, 98*, 232–237. doi:10.1136/archdischild-2012-302852

Hinks, A., Moncrieffe, H., & Martin, P. (2011). Association of the 5-aminoimidazole-4-caroxamide ribonucleotide transformylase gene with response to methotrexate in juvenile idiopathic arthritis. *Annals of Rheumatological Disease, 70*, 1395–1400.

Howington, L., Riddlesperger, K., & Cheek, D. (2011). Essential nursing competencies for genetics and genomics: Implications for critical care. *Critical Care Nurse, 31*(5), e1–e7. doi:10.4037/ccn2011867

Joly, Y., Sillon, G., Silverstein, T., Krajinovic, M., & Avard, D. (2008). Pharmacogenomics: Don't forget about the children. *Current Pharmacogenomics and Personalized Medicine, 6*, 77–84.

Kieling, C., Genro, J., Hutz, M., & Rohde, L. (2010). A current update on ADHD pharmacogenomics. *Pharmacogenomics, 11*(3), 407–419. doi:10.2217/PGS.10.28

Krajinovic, M., Lemieux-Blanchard, E., Chiasson, S., Primeau, M., Costea, I., & Moghrabi, A. (2004). Role of polymorphisms in MTHFR and MTHFD1 genes in the outcome of childhood acute lymphoblastic leukemia. *Pharmacogenomics Journal, 4*(1), 66–72.

Lee, J., Kang, H., Choi, J., Kim, N., Jang, M., Yeo, C., . . . Ahm, H. (2013). Pharacogenetic study of deferasirox, an iron chelating agent. *PLoS One, 8*(5), 364114. doi:10.1371/journal.pone.006414

Leeder, J. (2003). Developmental and pediatric pharmacogenomics. *Pharmacogenomics 4*, 331–341.

Leeder, J. (2004). Translating pharmacogenetics and pharmacogenomics into drug development for clinical pediatrics and beyond. *Drug Discovery Today, 9*(13), 567–573.

Leeder, J. & Kearns, G. (2012). Interpreting pharmacogenetic data in the developing neonate: The challenge of hitting a moving target. *Clinical Pharmacology Therapy, 92*(4), 434–436. doi:10.1038/clpt.2012.130

Leeder, J., Lantos, J., & Spielberg, S. (2010). Conference scene: Pediatric pharmacogenomics and personalized medicine. *Pharmacogenomics, 11*(12), 1691–1702. doi:10.2217/pgs.10.175

L'Huillier, A., Ing Lorenzini, K., Crisinel, P., Rebsamen, M., Fluss, J., Korff, C., . . . Desmeules, J. (2011). ABCB1 polymorphisms and neuropsychiatric adverse events in oseltamivir-treated children during influenza H1N1/09 pandemia. *Pharmacogenomics, 12*(10), 1493–1501. doi:10.2217/pgs.11.91

Manickaraj, A., & Mital, S. (2012). Personalized medicine in pediatric cardiology: Do little changes make a big difference. *Current Opinions in Pediatrics, 24*(5), 584–591. doi:10.1097/MOP.0b013e328357a4ea

McCracken, J., Badashova, K., & Posey, D. (2014). Positive effects of methylphenidate on hyperactivity are moderated by monoaminergic gene variants in children with autism spectrum disorders. *The Pharmacogenomics Journal, 14*, 295–302.

Moran, C., Thornburg, C., & Barfield, R. (2011). Ethical considerations for pharmacogenomic testing in pediatric clinical care and research. *Pharmacogenomics, 12*(6), 889–895. doi:10.2217/pgs.10.216

Neville, K., Becker, M., Goldman, J., & Kearns, G. (2011). Developmental pharmacogenomics. *Paediatric Anesthesia, 21*(3), 255–265. doi:10.1111/j.1460-9592.2011.03533.x

Pinto, N., Cohn, S., & Dolan, M. (2012). Using germline genomics to individualize pediatric cancer treatments. *Clinical Cancer Research, 18*(10), 2791–2800. doi:10.1158/1078-0432.CCR-11-1938

Rassekh, S., Ross, C., Carleton, B., & Hayden, M. (2013). Cancer pharmacogenomics in children: Research initiatives and progress to date. *Pediatric Drugs, 15*, 71–81. doi:10.1007/s40272-013-0021-9

Rieder, M. (2012). New ways to detect adverse drug reactions in pediatrics. *Pediatric Clinics of North America, 59*, 1071–1092. doi:10.1016/j.pcl.2012.07.010

Russo, R., Capasso, M., Paolucci, P., & Iolascon, A. (2011). Pediatric pharmacogenetic and pharmacogenomics studies: The current state and future perspectives. *European Journal of Clinical Pharmacology, 67*(Suppl 1), S17–S27. doi:10.1007/s00228-010-0931-1

Semsei, A., Erdelyi, D., & Ungvari, I. (2012). ABCC1 polymorphisms in anthracycline cardiotoxicity in childhood acute lymphoblastic leukemia. *Cellular Biology International, 36,* 79–86.

Shord, S., Thompson, D. M., Krempl, G. A., & Hanigan, M. H. (2006). Effect of concurrent medications on cisplatin-induced nephrotoxicity in patients with head and neck cancer. *Anticancer Drugs, 17*(2), 207–215.

Stevens, A., DeLeonibus, C., Hanson, D., Whatmore, A., Murray, P., Donn, R., . . . Clayton, P. (2013). Pediatric perspective on pharmacogenomics. *Pharmacogenomics, 14*(15), 1889–1905. doi:10.2217/PGS.13.193

Stockmann, C., Fassl, B., Gaedigk, R., Nkoy, F., Uchida, D., Monson, S., . . . Ward, R. (2013). Fluticasone propionate pharmacogenetics: CYP3A4*22 polymorphism and pediatric asthma control. *Journal of Pediatrics, 162*(6), 1222–1227. doi:10.1016/j.jpeds.2012.11.031

Szefler, S. (2003). Pediatric asthma: An approach to pharmacogenetics analysis. *Chest, 123*(Suppl 3), 434S–438S.

Tan-Kam, T., Suthisisang, C., Pavasuthipaisit, C., Limsila, P., Apichaya, P., & Sukasem, C. (2013). Importance of pharmacogenetics in the treatment of children with attention deficit hyperactive disorder: A case report. *Pharmacogenomics and Personalized Medicine, 6,* 3–7.

U.S. Food and Drug Administration, (2014). FDA's Sentinel Initiative. Retrieved from http://www.fda.gov/Safety/FDAsSentinelInitiative/default.htm

Visscher, H., Ross, C., & Rassekh, S. (2012). Canadian pharmacogenomics network for drug safety consortium. Pharmacogenomic prediction of anthracycline-induced cardiotoxicity in children. *Journal of Clinical Oncology, 30*(13), 1422–1428.

Wade, C., Tarini, B., & Wilfond, B. (2010). Growing up in the genomic era: Implications of whole-genome sequencing for children, families, and pediatric practice. *Annual Review of Genomics and Human Genetics, 14,* 535–555. doi:10.1146/annure-genom-091212-153425

Ward, R, Tammara, B., Sullivan, S., Stewart, D., Rath, N., Meng, X., . . . Comer, G. (2010). Single-dose, multiple-dose, and population pharmacokinetics of pantoprazole in neonates and preterm infants with a clinical diagnosis of gastroesophageal reflux disease (GERD). *European Journal of Clinical Pharmacology, 66*(6), 555–61.

Weinshilboum, R., & Sladek, S. (1980). Mercaptopurine pharmacogenetics: Monogenic inheritance of erythrocyte thiopurine methyltransferase activity. *American Journal of Human Genetics, 32,* 651–662.

Windsor, R., Strauss, S., Kallis, C., Wood, N., & Whelan, J. (2012). Germline genetic polymorphisms may influence chemotherapy response and disease outcome in osteosarcoma. *Cancer, 118*(7), 1856–1867. doi:10.1002/cncr.26472

Yang, J., Cheng, C., Devidas, M., Cao, X., Fan, Y., Campana, D., . . . Relling, M. (2011). Ancestry and pharmacogenomics of relapse in acute lymphoblastic leukemia, *National Genetics, 43*(3), 237–41. doi:10.1038/ng.763

Yang, J., Cheng, C., Yang, W., Pei, D., Cao, X., Fan, Y., . . . Relling, M. (2009). Genome-wide interrogation of germline genetic variation associated with treatment response in childhood acute lymphoblastic leukemia. *Journal of the American Medical Association, 301*(4), 393–403. doi: 10.1001/jama.2009.7

Pharmacogenomics and Older Adult Patients

Dennis J. Cheek, PhD, RN, FAHA

7

The growing population of older adults will not only have an effect on the already strained healthcare system but also on all healthcare providers, especially nurses. Of course, many older adults will have normal physiological changes related to the processes of aging but also will present with common pathophysiological responses requiring pharmacological treatment. The nurses of the future will have to draw upon their traditional educational preparation, including pharmacotherapeutics, as well as the growing field of pharmacogenomics and its effect on the clinical practice of older adults. Nurses will be part of clinical practice and research that is driven by the promise of individualized drug therapy to maximize drug efficacy and minimize drug toxicity.

This chapter will discuss the roles and responsibilities of entry-level and advanced practice nurses in pharmacogenomics and older adult patients. The discussion will provide an overview of the growing older adult population, physiological changes related to age that affect pharmacokinetics and pharmacodynamics, and medication therapy management, along with common adverse drug reactions and the use of pharmacogenomics to target specific disease markers, improve likelihood of response, and enhance drug safety in the older adult population (McCarthy, McLeod, & Ginsburg, 2013).

OBJECTIVES

- Pharmacogenomics is important in avoiding drug-drug interactions in older adults who are often taking multiple medications.
- The identification of specific drug metabolism enzymes involved in drug metabolism will impact the older adult's drug regimen given the higher prevalence of comorbidity.
- Pharmacogenomics will reduce adverse drug reactions experienced by the older adult.

An Increasing Older Adult Population

The American population is living longer and getting older. The proportion of men and women over the age of 65 is growing, as noted by the U.S. Census Bureau 2010 Census Report (U.S. Census Bureau, 2011). This increase of older adults does not take into account the Baby Boomers, who are currently age 50–68 and are contributing to the population of older adults age 65 and up. See Figure 7.1.

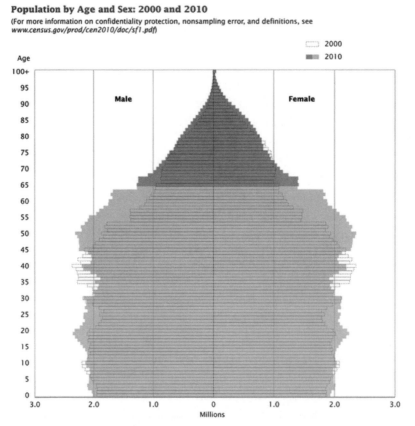

Figure 7.1   Growing Population by Age and Sex. U.S. Census Bureau, Census 2000 Summary File 1 and 2010 Census Summary File 1 (U.S. Census Bureau, 2010).

A June 2012 report by the Federal Interagency Forum on Aging-Related Statistics (http://www.agingstats.gov) noted that if the average American survives to age 65, he or she could expect to live another 19.2 years. The Federal Interagency Forum on Aging-Related Statistics report also noted that if the average American woman reaches age 85, she would live an additional 7 years on average; and the American male who reaches age 85 would live an additional 5.9 years on average.

The older adult population is an important and growing segment of the United States population. The U.S. Census Bureau reported in the 2010 census that between 2000 and 2010, the older adult population age 65 years and older grew at a faster rate (15.7%) than did the total United States population (9.7%). During this same time, the number of males older than age 65 also grew at a significant rate, to the point of reducing the gap between men and women age 65. As the population of men and women who reach age 65 continues to grow, we know that on average, they have an additional 19.2 years of life expectancy. There are growing implications for this group of older adults with regard to not only the social and economic factors within society, but also family dynamics, which may also involve caregiving. With individual older adults, there are also implications specifically focused on the normal physiological or pathophysiological changes that lead to chronic disease (requiring pharmacological management) and eventual mortality.

Leading Causes of Death

The top five leading causes of death of older adults in 2011 were heart disease, malignant neoplasms, chronic lower respiratory diseases, cerebrovascular disease, and Alzheimer's disease (Hoyert & Xu, 2012). According to the same authors, the next five leading causes of death are diabetes, influenza and pneumonia, nephritis, suicide, and septicemia. These leading causes of death in the older adult population have also been reported by men and women age 65 or older as chronic health conditions (Federal Interagency Forum on Aging-Related Statistics, 2012). These reported chronic health conditions include heart disease, hypertension, cerebrovascular disease, asthma, chronic bronchitis or emphysema, neoplasms, diabetes, and arthritis (Federal Interagency Forum on Aging-Related Statistics, 2012).

Polypharmacy and Seniors

During the same period (2011), the top 10 prescriptions were hydrocodone/acetaminophen, simvastatin, lisinopril, levothyroxine sodium, amlodipine besylate, omeprazole, azithromycin, amoxicillin, metformin, and hydrochlorothiazide (IMS Institute for Healthcare Informatics, 2011). In the pharmacological management of older adults with chronic disease, even though older adults make up only 13% of the population, they account for 34% of all prescription medication use and 40% of all over-the-counter (OTC) medication use (Ferrini & Ferrini, 2012). The Agency for Healthcare Research and Quality (AHRQ), in its May 2009 statistical brief (www.ahrq.gov), noted that as of 2006, the average older adult used approximately six prescriptions, which was an increase from five, noted in the past decade. This report also documents that the number of prescriptions per person increases with age (Stagnitti, 2009). With increasing age and potential of chronic disease is the possibility of increasing need for pharmacological management of said chronic disease.

Polypharmacy

The increase in number of prescriptions, which also increases with age, is *polypharmacy*, from the Greek *poly* (many) and *pharmakon* (drug). Polypharmacy can also cause harm or adverse drug reactions for the older adult (Masoodi, 2008).

The harm or adverse drug reactions (ADRs) caused by polypharmacy are responsible for numerous unnecessary costs both to the healthcare system at large and the patient: in this case, the older adult (Budnitz, Lovegrove, & Shehab, 2011). An estimated 2,216,000 hospitalized patients experience serious ADRs; and of these patients, 106,000 die annually from an ADR (Lazarou, Pormeranz, & Corey, 1998). To place these numbers in perspective: If included in the Centers for Disease Control and Prevention (CDC) rankings of causes of death, deaths from ADRs would rank as the fifth leading cause of death annually within the United States (Centers for Disease Control and Prevention, 2012).

In older adult patients, as many as 30% of persons admitted to the hospital are admitted for medication-related problems (MRP; Marcum et al., 2012). In the nursing home setting, for every $1 USD spent on drugs, $1.33 in healthcare resources are consumed to treat medication-related problems (Bootman, Harrison, & Cox, 1997). The risk of ADRs rises exponentially with the addition of each new medication to an older adult's drug regimen. Despite this, the healthcare system is increasing concomitant use of medication each year (Denham, 1990).

In addition, the more medication(s) that an older adult is taking concurrently, the higher is the risk for an ADR. Individual medications have their own side effects or ADRs. Another drug prescribed to the older adult to counter side effects or an ADR can lead to what is described as a "prescribing cascade" (Antimisaris & Cheek, 2014). For an older adult, this cascade can be caused by seeing numerous healthcare providers. The average number of healthcare providers seen by a person older than age 65 is seven (Antimisaris & Cheek, 2014).

Another risk factor is the advent of online and mail-order pharmacies, as well as the plethora of large chain pharmacies, resulting in the older adult filling prescriptions at multiple pharmacies versus one primary pharmacy. A nurse can encourage patients to use a pharmacy that can check patient records chain-wide to reduce the risk of polypharmacy. The other beneficial effect of a single pharmacy nationwide is that older adults who travel would be able to walk into the chain pharmacy anywhere and have the prescription refilled.

Pharmacokinetics

The normal aging process of the older adult has an effect on all aspects of the pharmacokinetic processes of absorption, distribution, metabolism, and excretion. Even in the absence of specific chronic diseases, the normal aging process is associated with changes in muscle, gastrointestinal (GI) tract, and liver and kidney function that affect pharmacokinetics (Aymanns, Keller, Maus, Hartmann, & Czock, 2010). Reduction in the total body water with corresponding increases in total body fat will have an effect upon volume of distribution (Vd; Fulop, Worum, Csongor, Foris, & Leovey, 1985). Increasing age usually reduces GI motility, and blood flow and gastric acid secretion are reduced. The net effect of all these changes makes it difficult to predict the variations in drug absorption in the older adult that are generally considered to be minimal (Hutchinson & O'Brien, 2007; Mangoni & Jackson, 2004).

Increase in age also usually results in a corresponding reduction in liver volume and blood flow, with a corresponding reduction in metabolic reactions—in particular, those that are collectively known as *Phase 1*, which are the reactions catalyzed by the cyto-chrome 450 (CYP450) enzymes, which may lead to reduction of drug clearance (Mangoni & Jackson, 2004; Zoli et al., 1999). With increasing age, there is also a loss of renal paren-chyma as well as decrease in renal plasma flow, which results in a progressive decline in glomerular filtration rate (GFR). This decline in GFR is also associated with age-related increase in the half-life of many drugs fall under first-order elimination (Coresh & Astor, 2006; Musso, Macias Nunez, & Oreopoulos, 2007).

Katzung and Trevor (2013) state, "Drugs with first-order elimination have a charac-teristic half-life elimination that is constant regardless of the amount of drug in the body. The concentration of such a drug in the blood will decrease by 50% for every half-life. Most drugs in clinical use demonstrate first-order kinetics."

Pharmacodynamics

The normal physiological aging process in the older adult not only affects pharmacoki-netics but also pharmacodynamics. These changes include receptor number and affinity, as well as signal transduction. The end results may manifest in increased sensitivity to the effect of a specific drug as well as the potential to decrease responsiveness of the receptor to a specific drug (Delafuente, 2008; Hutchinson & O'Brien, 2007).

The central nervous system (CNS) and cardiovascular system are the two specific sys-tems most significantly affected with pharmacodynamics alterations. Examples of chang-es to be encountered include the CNS, where alteration in the gamma-aminobutyric acid (GABA) neurotransmission increases sensitivity by the older adult to benzodiazepines, including ADR (El Desoky, 2007; Hutchinson & O'Brien, 2007).

The acetylcholine neurotransmission system is also affected with age. There is a de-crease in the number of cholinergic neurons, decrease in choline uptake by the neuron, reduced choline acetyltransferase, increased acetylcholinesterase and corresponding re-duction in the cholinergic receptors, all resulting in increased sensitivity to anticholiner-gic drugs (El Desoky, 2007; Hutchinson & O'Brien, 2007). The number of dopamine type 2 receptors increases in the aging brain, increasing the chance of delirium in an older adult who takes anticholinergic or dopaminergic drugs. There is also a decrease in the number of dopaminergic neurons in the substantia nigra, which will increase the likeli-hood that the older adult will experience extrapyramidal side effects from antidopami-nergic drugs (El Desoky, 2007; Hutchinson & O'Brien, 2007).

ADR is a multifactorial and complex problem involving alterations in the pharmacokinetics and pharmacodynamics. Thus, we must ask whether there is a connection with the older adult underlying genomic makeup and pharmacology or pharmacogenomics.

Pharmacogenomics

Pharmacogenomics is a broad field of study that seeks to understand the role that human genetic variation across the entire genome plays in disease susceptibility and progression, as well as the role human genetic variation plays in determining treatment options and drug response. Pharmacogenetics is a subset of pharmacogenomics, concerned specifically with using DNA and amino acid sequence data to inform drug development, testing, efficacy, and safety.

> SNPs are substitutions of a single base in the nucleotide sequence.

One important application of pharmacogenetics is correlating individual genetic variation with drug responses (NHGRI, 2014). The cellular expression and function of transporters, metabolizing enzymes, and specific receptors depend in part on genetic factors that with today's technologies can be assessed in patients. These factors, which are different types of inherited genetic variants, include deletion, insertions, and the multiplication or repetition of specific sequences involving large portions of DNA. The most frequent and common genetic variant identified and tested with regard to pharmacogenetics is single nucleotide polymorphisms (SNPs; NHGRI, 2014). Studies of the human genome sequence have established that there are more than 15 million SNPs, some of which are benign (such as hair and eye color) or as pathological as development of sickle cell anemia or alteration of specific drug effects (NCBI-SNP, 2014).

The implications of pharmacogenomics on nursing practice are significant. No longer will drugs be prescribed for the general public, but a specific drug will be used for the specific patient genotype, resulting in personalized medicine. The Federal Drug Administration (FDA) has a growing list ($n = 113$) of drugs with pharmacogenomics implications for targeting specific drug therapy, avoiding ADRs, and optimizing drug doses (FDA, 2014).

Targeting Drug Therapy

One of the most high-profile diseases to benefit from our understanding of pharmacogenomics is cancer, with targeting of specific pharmacological therapies. The exemplar is discovery of the HER-2, which is a biomarker overexpressed in about 30% of breast cancer patients and associated with an increase of adverse outcomes (Slamon et al., 1987). The 1998 development of trastuzumab (Herceptin), a humanized monoclonal antibody that targets the HER-2 biomarker and reduces adverse outcomes, is a significant achievement. Standard testing for HER-2 in now baseline in the workup and management of breast cancer (Ross et al., 2009). Pharmacogenomics is revolutionizing cancer treatment as genomic technologies allow for the refining of tumor types to allow for truly individualized therapies.

Avoiding Adverse Drug Reactions

Other implications of pharmacogenomics in nursing practice include the ADR associated with the HLA-B*5701 genotype for the HIV drug abacavir (Mallal et al., 2008), which leads to a hypersensitivity reaction of a multiorgan syndrome characterized by two or more clinical signs or symptoms that can include fever, rash, GI, and respiratory symptoms. In another example, the HLA-B*1502 genotype for the antiseizure drug carbamazepine results in adverse reaction, such as Stevens-Johnson Syndrome or toxic epidermal necrolysis (TEN), which are two forms of life-threatening skin conditions in which cell death causes the epidermis to separate from the dermis (Chung et al., 2004). Bedside and advanced practice nurses need to be aware of the carriers of these specific genotypes so as to avoid the drug entirely and eliminate specific serious ADRs.

Additionally, the FDA has put forth FDA Alerts that support the recommendation of pretherapy screening for the presence of HLA-B alleles. Genetic testing for HLA-B*5701 is currently available, and all patients should be screened for the HLA-B*5701 allele before starting abacavir or abacavir-containing medications. Avoidance of abacavir therapy in HLA-B*5701 positive patients will significantly reduce the risk of developing hypersensitivity reaction.

Optimizing Drug Doses

Pharmacogenomics should also be used in adjusting doses of warfarin (Coumadin) based upon the CYP2C9 genotype (liver metabolism enzyme) and VKORC1 genotype (Vitamin K epoxide reductase enzyme) to improve efficacy and reduce ADRs (Aithal, Day,

Kesteven, & Daily, 1999; Rost et al., 2004). CYP2C9*1 is the hepatic enzyme responsible for metabolizing S-warfarin, which is three to five times more potent than R-warfarin.

> S-warfarin and R-warfarin are enantiomers, or mirror images, of the warfarin molecule.

The genetic *polymorphisms* (variations) CYP2C9*2 and CYP2C9*3, which are common in the general population, result in decreased clearance and increased blood levels of S-warfarin (Jorgensen, FitzGerald, Oyee, Pirmohamed, & Williamson, 2012). Warfarin inhibits VKOR, which is encoded by the VKORC1 gene. Variations within this gene also affect the patient's response to warfarin. The major variation in the VKORC1 gene is the1639GA genotype, which decreases the expression of VKOR. Patients with this genotype are susceptible to inhibition by warfarin, so the warfarin dosage should be reduced (International Warfarin Pharmacogenetics Consortium, 2009).

Pharmacogenomics is also used in drug efficacy with the antiplatelet agent clopidogrel (Plavix) and specific CYP2C19 variants that alter the conversion of the prodrug clopidogrel to an active metabolite (Holmes, Perel, Shah, Hingorani, & Casas, 2011). The specific cytochromes enzymes CYP2C9 and CYP2C19 are involved in the anticoagulant and antiplatelet agents.

The cytochrome enzyme CYP2D6 is responsible for approximately 25% of all drugs biotransformed in the liver, including many of the antidepressants and antipsychotic agents. The variant CYP2D6*1 allele is responsible for extensive (primary) metabolism of many drugs. This hepatic metabolizing enzyme has 90 known variants that slow drug metabolism, increasing serum drug concentrations. In the extreme case, for patients with the allele CYP2D6*4, the expressed protein is inactive, so serum drug levels increase dramatically (Kirchheiner et al., 2003). Conversely, the variant CYP2D6*2 increases enzyme activity, decreasing serum drug levels.

Practice Resources

In the clinical practice of caring for older adults at the bedside, the new science of the patient's genetic makeup and its interaction with pharmacology is *pharmacogenomics*. To accommodate this new and growing field of pharmacogenomics with the ever rapidly escalating genetic information and pharmacology, a Pharmacogenomics Knowledgebase (PharmGKB.org) has been established to assist the practicing nurse (Whirl-Carrillo et al., 2012). The basic foundation of this new knowledge base, PharmGKB, is the primary literature on pharmacogenetics and pharmacogenomics. This primary literature is reviewed, categorized, analyzed, and integrated into a form of gene variant annotation. PharmGKB not only provides pharmacogenomics knowledge but also the clinical implementation of such knowledge. PharmGKB is involved in development of knowledge base, data sharing, and establishment of consortiums, such as the Clinical Pharmacogenetics Implementation Consortium (CPIC), which was formed in late 2009 between PharmGKB and the Pharmacogenomic Research Network (CPIC, 2014; PharmGKB.org, 2014). The CPIC genotype and dosing guidelines are peer-reviewed and published in *Clinical Pharmacology & Therapeutics* with simultaneous posting in PharmGKB.

The CPIC (www.pharmgkb.org/page/cpic) has provided specific drug dosing guidelines for a growing list of drugs. The following list was current when this book published:

- abacavir
- allopurinol
- amitriptyline
- azathioprine
- boceprevir
- capecitabine
- carbamazepine
- clomipramine
- clopidogrel
- codeine
- desipramine
- doxepin
- fluorouracil
- imipramine
- ivacaftor
- mercaptopurine
- nortriptyline
- peginterferon alfa-2a
- peginterferon alfa-2b
- phenytoin
- rasburicase
- ribavirin
- simvastatin
- tegafur
- telaprevir
- thioguanine
- trimipramine
- warfarin

Internationally, the Saw Swee Hock School of Public Health; National University of Singapore (NUS); Health Science Authority, Singapore (HSA); and Genome Institute of Singapore (GIS) have developed the Singapore Pharmacogenomics Portal (NUS, 2014). The Singapore Pharmacogenomics Portal (SPP) is an integration of information from four separate databases (NUS, 2014):

- **PharmGKB (www.pharmgkb.org):** Integrated resource about how variation in human genetics leads to variation in response to drugs.
- **Drug Bank (www.drugbank.ca):** A Canadian public resource on drug chemistry, interaction, pharmacology, interaction, metabolism, and action.
- **International HapMap (www.hapmap.org):** The International HapMap Project is a partnership of scientists and funding agencies from Canada, China, Japan, Nigeria, the United Kingdom, and the United States to develop a public resource that will help researchers find genes associated with human disease and response to pharmaceuticals.
- **Singapore Genetic Variation Project (SGVP; www.statgen.nus.edu. sg/~SPGx/SPGx_intro.php):** This project aims to characterize the extent of common variation in the human genome across at least 1 million single nucleotide polymorphisms (SNPs) for DNA samples from each of the three ethnic groups in Singapore—Chinese, Malays, and Indians.

SPP should make it easier for researchers and regulators to compare genetic variation across populations for genetic variants that affect drug responses, dosages, and adverse drug reactions (NUS, 2014).

Another free resource available to the clinician is the website WarfarinDosing.org. This website is developed and supported by Barnes-Jewish Hospital at Washington University Medical Center and the National Institutes of Health (NIH). This website provides recommendations for the initial doses of warfarin based upon the genetic information for two specific genes: cytochrome P450 2C9 (CYP2C9) and vitamin K epoxide reductase (VKORC1; WarfarinDosing.org, 2014).

Here are additional resources available to the clinician:

- **Genelex YouScript (Genelex.com):** This laboratory resource is a new way of using genetic tests and knowledge of drug metabolism to personalize the patient's therapeutic responses to his or her medication regimen. The current DNA test panel covers all the clinically significant genetic variants in CYP2D6, CYP2C9, CYP2C19, and VKORC1, as well as providing pharmacists personalized prescription plans for challenging patients (Genelex.com, 2014).

- **The Spartan RX (www.spartanbio.com):** This FDA–approved point-of-care device assesses for the presence of the common genetic variants of the *CYP2C19* gene. The product of this specific gene is responsible for the conversion of the antiplatelet agent clopidogrel from a prodrug to an active drug. Approximately one in three patients has this variant (Spartan, 2014). This device has the ability to take a collection, such as a buccal swab sample that is placed into a predesigned tube, and then the sample/tube is placed into the Spartan RX device with results in 60 minutes. The results will indicate either no variant in CYP2C19 or that a genetic variant is present in the CYP2C19 gene.

Educational Resources

There are numerous resources available to the nurse to assist in knowledge acquisition and understanding pharmacogenomics at the bedside:

- **National Genetic and Genomics Education Centre (www.geneticseducation.nhs.uk):** Funded and established by the National Health Service of United Kingdom in 2005, the centre is working with both healthcare professionals and patients, with the key aim of providing leadership in genetic education, raising awareness, involving patients and families in genetic decisions, and facilitating genetic/genomics into curricula (National Health Service of United Kingdom, 2014).

- **The Pharmacogenomics Education Program (https://pharmacogenomics.ucsd. edu):** This is an evidence-based program bridging the gap between science and practice. The PharmGenEd program was initially supported by a grant from the Centers for Disease Control and Prevention in 2008–2012. The program has continued to be supported by the University of California San Diego Skaggs School of Pharmacy and Pharmaceutical Sciences in collaboration with national pharmacy, medical, and healthcare organizations to deliver the PharmGenEd material to healthcare providers nationwide (PharmGenEd.org, 2014).

- **Genetics/Genomics Competency Center Education Center (G2C2; www.g-2-c-2.org):** G2C2 was initially funded by the National Human Genome Research Institute (NHGRI). The University of Virginia built the initial web-based architecture for G2C2 and now continues with ongoing funding from NHGRI. The mission of G2C2 is to provide high-quality education resources for group instruction or self-directed learning for genetic counselors, nurses, physician assistants, and pharmacists. In the website pharmacist section is a growing list of resources related to the application of pharmacogenomics to practice (G2C2.org, 2014).

Summary

As part of providing high-quality care to the older adult patient, the nurse is involved with the medication therapy. With the completion of the Human Genome Project, there has been a significant growth of genetic/genomic knowledge being translated into drug therapy (PharmGKB.org). Nurses of the future will not only need to review drug information sheets but also lab data, including genetic/genomic profiles of their patient prior to the administration of prescribed medication. The nurse is in the ideal position to implement the pharmacogenomics principles and to assist in the targeting of specific medications, avoiding ADRs, and optimizing drug dosing, thus increasing drug efficacy in his or her patient. With pharmacogenomics testing and a comprehensive understanding of the variables and science, the nurse will be able to provide therapy and support as well as accurately collect data from ongoing therapeutic drug monitoring.

Questions

Warfarin labeling now includes dosing recommendations for which two genotypes?

    a.   CYP2C19*1 and VKOR

    b.   1639GA and VKOR

    c.   CYP2C9 and VKORC1 *

    d.   CYP2D6 and CYP2D6*1

The FDA recommends genetic testing for patients with HIV before they are prescribed which of the following drugs?

    a.   abacavir *

    b.   atazanavir

    c.   indinavir

    d.   ritonavir

Critical Thinking Question: Clopidogrel has just been ordered for your patient. What are the specific pharmacogenomics implications?

Key Points

- Pharmacogenomics in the older adult is important in targeting specific drug therapy.

- Using pharmacogenomics testing will reduce ADRs encountered by older adult.

- Increasing usage of pharmacogenomics testing will increase drug optimization and efficacy for the older adult.

References

Aithal, G. P., Day, C. P., Kesteven, P. J., & Daly, A. K. (1999). Association of polymorphisims in the cyto-chrome P450 CY2C9 with warfarin dose requirement and risk of bleeding complications. *Lancet, 353,* 717–719.

Antimisaris, D., & Cheek, D. J. (2014). Polypharmacy. In K. Mauk, (Ed.), *Gerontological Nursing: Competencies for care* (417–456). Burlington, MA: Jones & Bartlett Learning.

Aymanns, C., Keller, F., Maus, S., Hartmann, B., & Czock, D. (2010). Review on pharmacokinetics and pharmacodynamics and the aging kidney. *Clinical Journal of the American Society of Nephrology, 5,* 314–327.

Bootman, J. L., Harrison, D. L., & Cox, E. (1997). The health care cost of drug-related morbidity and mortality in nursing facilities. *Archive of Internal Medicine, 157,* 2089–2096.

Budnitz, D. S., Lovegrove, M. C., & Shehab, N. (2011). Emergency hospitalizations for adverse drug events in older Americans. *New England Journal of Medicine, 365*(21), 2002–2012.

Centers for Disease Control and Prevention (CDC). (2012). Retrieved from http://www.cdc.gov

Chung, W. H., Hung, S. I., Hong, H. S., Hsih, M. S., Yang, L. C., Ho, H. C., . . . Chen, Y. T. (2004). Medical genetics: A marker for Steven-Johnson syndrome. *Nature, 428,* 486.

Coresh, J. & Astor, B. (2006). Decreased kidney function in the elderly: clinical and preclinical, neither benign. *Annals of Internal Medicine, 145,* 299–301.

CPIC. (2014). Retrieved from http://www.pharmgkb.org/page/cpic

Delafuente, J. C. (2008). Pharmacokinetic and pharmacodynamic alterations in the geriatric patient. *The Consultant Pharmacist, 23,* 324–334.

Denham, M. J. (1990). Adverse drug reactions. *British Medical Bulletin, 46,* 53–62.

El Desoky, E. S. (2007). Pharmacokinetic-pharmacodynamic crisis in the elderly. *American Journal of Therapeutics 14,* 488–498.

Food & Drug Administration (FDA). (2014). Retrieved from http://www.fda.gov

Federal Interagency Forum on Aging-Related Statistics. (June 2012). Older Americans 2012: Key indicators of well-being. Federal Interagency Forum on Aging-Related Statistics. Washington, DC: U.S. Government Printing Office.

Ferrini, A, & Ferrini, R. (2012). *Health in the later years* (5th ed). Boston, MA: McGraw Hill.

Fulop, T., Jr., Worum, I., Csongor, J., Foris, G., & Leovey, A. (1985). Body composition in elderly people. I. Determination of body composition by multiisotope method and the elimination kinetics of these isotopes in healthy elderly subjects. *Gerontology, 31,* 6–14.

G2C2.org. (2014). *About the project.* Retrieved from http://www.g-2-c-2.org

Genelex.com. (2014). *YouScript.* Retrieved from http://www.youscript.com

Holmes, M. V., Perel, P., Shah, T., Hingorani, A. D., & Casas, J. P. (2011). CYP2C19 genotype, clopidogrel metabolism, platelet function, and cardiovascular events: A systematic review and meta-analysis. *Journal of the American Medical Association, 306,* 2704–2714.

Hoyert, D. L., & Xu, J. Q. (2012). Deaths: Preliminary data for 2011. National vital statistics reports, *61*(6). Hyattsville, MD: National Center for Health Statistics.

Hutchinson, L. C., & O'Brien, C. E. (2007). Changes in pharmacokinetics and pharmacodynamics in the elderly patient. *Journal of Pharmacy Practice, 20,* 4–12.

IMS Institute for Healthcare Informatics. (April 2011). The Use of Medicines in the United States: Review of 2010. Parsippany, NJ: Author.

International Warfarin Pharmacogenetics Consortium. (2009). Estimation of the warfarin dose with clinical and pharmacogenetic data. *New England Journal of Medicine, 360*(8), 753–764.

Jorgensen, A. L., FitzGerald, R. J., Oyee, J., Pirmohamed, M., & Williamson, P. R. (2012). Influence of CYP2C9 and VKORC1 on patient response to warfarin: a systematic review and meta-analysis. *PLoS ONE, 7*(8):e44064. doi: 10.1371/journal.pone.0044064

Kirchheiner, J., Muller, G., Meinke, I., Wernecke, K. D., Roots, I. & Brockmoller, J. (2003). Effects of polymorphisms in CYP2D6, CYP2C9, and CYP2C19 on trimipramine pharmacokinetics. *Journal of Clinical Psychopharmacology, 23,* 459–466.

Lazarou, J., Pomeranz, B. H., & Corey, P. N. (1998). Incidence of adverse drug reactions in hospitalized patients. *Journal of the American Medical Association, 279,* 1200–1205.

Mallal, S., Phillips, E., Carosi, G., Molina, J. M., Workman, C., Tomazic, J., . . . Benbow, A. (2008). PREDICT-1 study team, HLA-*B5701 screening to hypersensitivity to abacavir. *New England Journal of Medicine, 358,* 568–579.

Mangoni, A. A., & Jackson, S. H. (2004). Age-related changes in pharmacokinetics and pharmacodynamics: Basic principles and practical applications. *British Journal of Clinical Pharmacology, 57,* 6–14

Marcum, Z. A., Amuan, M. E., Hanlon, J. T., Aspinall, S. L., Handler, S. M., Ruby, C. M., & Pugh, M. J. (2012). Prevalence of unplanned hospitalizations caused by adverse drug reactions in older veterans. *Journal of the American Geriatric Society, 60*(1), 34–41.

Masoodi, N. A. (2008). Polypharmacy: To err is human, to correct divine. *British Journal of Medical Practioners, 1*(1), 6–9.

McCarthy, J. J., McLeod, H. L. & Ginsburg, G. S. (2013). Genomic medicine: a decade of successes, challenges and opportunities. *Science & Translational Medicine.* 5, 189sr4.

Musso, C. G., Macias Nunez, J. F., & Oreopoulos, D. G. (2007). Physiological similarities and differences between renal aging and chronic renal disease. *Journal of Nephrology, 20,* 586–587.

National Center for Biotechnology Information (NCBI)-SNP Database. (2014). Retrieved from http://www.ncbi.nlm.nih.gov/snp

National Health Service of United Kingdom. (2014). *National genetics and genomics education centre.* Retrieved from http://www.geneticseducation.nhs.uk

National Human Genome Research Institute [NHGRI]. (2014). Retrieved from http://www.genome.gov/

National University of Singapore [NUS] (2014). Retrieved from http://www.nus.edu.sg/

PharmGenEd.org. (2014). *Overview of PharmGenEd.* Retrieved from https://pharmacogenomics.ucsd.edu

PharmGKB.org. (2014). *Overview of PharmGKB.* Retrieved from https://www.pharmgkb.org

Ross, J. S., Slodkowska, E. A., Symmans, W. F., Pusztai, L., Ravidin, P. M. & Hortobagyi, G. N. (2009). The HER-2 receptor and breast cancer: Ten years of targeted anti-HER-2 therapy and personalized medicine. *Oncologist, 14,* 320–368.

Rost, S., Fregin, A., Ivaskevicius, V., Conzelmann, E., Hortnagel, K., Pelz, H. J., . . . Oldenburg, J. (2004). Mutations in VKORC1 cause warfarin resistance and multiple coagulation factor deficiency type 2. *Nature, 427,* 537–541.

Singapore Pharmacogenomics Portal. (2014). Retrieved from http://www.statgen.nus.edu.sg/~SPGx/SPGx_intro.php

Slamon, D. J., Clark, G. M., Wong, S. G., Levin, W. J., Ullrich, A., & McQuire, W. L. (1987). Human breast cancer: Correlation of relapse and survival with amplification of HER-2/neu oncogene. *Science, 235,* 177–182.

Spartan. (2014). *Spartan RX.* Retrieved from http://www.spartanbio.com

Stagnitti, M. N. (2009). Average number of total (including refills) and unique prescriptions by select person characteristics, 2006. Retrieved from http://www.meps.ahrq.gov/mepsweb/data files/publications/st245/stat245.pdf

U.S. Census Bureau. (November 2011). The Older Population 2010. 2010 Census Brief. Washington, DC: U.S. Government Printing Office.

WarfarinDosing.org. (2014). *Warfarin dosing.* Retrieved from http://www.warfindosing.org

Whirl-Carrillo, M., McDonagh, E. M., Hebert, J. M., Gong, L., Sangkuhl, K., Thorn, C. F., . . . Klein, T. E. (2012). Pharmacogenomics for personalized medicine. *Clinical Pharmacology & Therapeutics, 92*(4), 414–417.

Zoli, M., Magalotti, D., Bianchi, G., Gueli, C., Orlandini, C., Grimaldi, M., & Marchesini, G. (1999). Total and functional hepatic blood flow decrease in parallel with ageing. *Age and Ageing, 28,* 29–33.

Influence of Pharmacogenomics on Patients– Oncology

8

Erika Santos, PhD, RN, MSc
Silvia Regina Secoli, PhD, RN, MSc

Antineoplastic treatment shows substantial variability in tumor response at the expense of considerable toxicity, which compromises the quality of life (QoL) of cancer patients. Often due to the consequences of treatment toxicity, treatment costs become even higher; therefore, it is imperative to use methods that allow the correct selection of appropriate therapeutic resources (Bertino, 2013; Crona & Innocenti, 2012).

The ability to associate DNA characteristics with drug response provides an individualized approach that has an important significance in clinical practice (Zdanowicz & American Society of Health-System Pharmacists, 2010). These pharmacogenomic markers may help to predict response to treatment and individualized regimens and to identify whether the patient will present a serious adverse reaction based on the genotype of the patient (Bertino, 2013; Crona & Innocenti, 2012). The objectives of this chapter are to classify pharmacogenetic predictors, address pharmacogenomic markers and their FDA drugs, and highlight key points that nurses should consider in the incorporation of personalized pharmacogenomics therapeutic strategy.

OBJECTIVES

- List the classification of pharmacogenomic predictors.
- Discuss the impact of germline variants on toxicity and response to cancer patients submitted to treatment with antineoplasic drugs.
- Describe how somatic changes can affect the choice of treatment in oncology.
- Describe the recommendations for pharmacogenomic care in patients undergoing treatment with antineoplastic drugs.

Pharmacogenetic Predictors

According to Hertz and McLeod (2013), pharmacogenetic predictors can be classified into four groups according to their purpose:

- **Predictors of toxicity:** Related to the individual's sensitivity to the drug and are located in the germline genome
- **Predictors of exposure:** Related to drug sensitivity and are located in the germline genome
- **Prognostic predictors:** Related to the tumor's behavior and may be located in the germline or somatic genome
- **Predictors of effectiveness:** Related to the sensitivity of the tumor to the drug and are located in the somatic genome

Tumor and germline changes are different. Tumor changes result in tumor variability and are associated with response to treatment. Comparatively, germline changes may account for patient variability, not only affecting the pharmacokinetics but also the pharmacodynamics of drugs and the risk of developing diseases (O'Donnell & Ratain, 2012).

Pharmacogenomic Markers

Pharmacogenomic markers may also be used to guide the dose prescription. It is clear that in oncology, the traditional method for setting the dose of an antineoplastic agent leads to the establishment of a single dose—not a range of doses. In this method, the calculation is based on body surface area, or even using the calculation of the area under the curve, which considers the glomerular filtration rate (GFR) and creatinine clearance. However, patients with defects in enzymes responsible for the metabolism of drugs exhibit severe toxicities even with drugs prescribed in standard doses. Also, some patients with high enzymatic activity present a risk of recurrence (Bertino, 2013; Crona & Innocenti, 2012). Therefore, predictors of toxicity and exposure can be used with benefits to patients.

In this chapter, we divide the pharmacogenomic markers into two aspects: germline variants and somatic variants. We will present a table with all drugs approved in oncology with the FDA pharmacogenomic markers.

Since the first reports (1950s) related to genetics, drug availability, and effects, an increase in the number of identified germline variants that affect not only the pharmacokinetics but also pharmacodynamics has been observed.

Germline Variants

Germline variations are changes in the DNA sequence that are inherited. These variations may include SNPs (single-nucleotide polymorphisms), insertions and deletions of one or a few nucleotides (indels), larger deletions and insertions, CNVs (copy number variations), VNTRs (variable number tandem repeats), and gene rearrangements. Whether a variation has a functional consequence depends on its location and nature (Bertino, 2013). Germline variations affect individual predisposition to cancer or disease progression. Although a significant part of the knowledge regarding cancer biology and development is derived from individuals that require cancer predisposition genetic testing, the results may not be representative for the general population (Hall et al., 2009).

Purine Analogs

Purine analogs, such as mercaptopurine (6-MP) and thioguanine (6-TG), are used to treat acute lymphoblastic leukemia (ALL). 6-MP and 6-TG are prodrugs that are activated by thioguanine nucleotides that are incorporated into DNA and RNA, causing DNA damage and cytotoxicity. TPMT (thiopurine S-methyltransferase) is an enzyme responsible for the inactivation of these drugs (Zdanowicz & American Society of Health-System Pharmacists, 2010). 6-MP is essential in the maintenance phase of ALL and has a narrow therapeutic window with the potential for serious toxicity, which is a result of the metabolism of the prodrug into its active metabolites in the cell (Appell et al., 2013).

6-MP is inactivated by TPMT to thiuric acid and oxidation to 6-methylmercaptopurine by xanthine oxidase. However, hematopoietic cells do not have measurable activity of xanthine oxidase, leaving the TPMT as the primary inactivating enzyme for 6-MP. In the absence or reduction of TPMT activity, 6-MP is metabolized to 6-TG, which has suppressive activity in the bone marrow (Bertino, 2013).

It is important to recognize that individuals have this change in the metabolism of 6-MP to prevent fatal bone marrow failure and ensure safe dosing.

Genetic variations in the TPMT gene have been identified. However, only three variants to date have a clinical impact (Bertino, 2013)—TPMT*2, *3A, and *3C, which represent 95% of the variants of the gene designated (Adam de Beaumais et al., 2011). The TPMT*2 variant is the result of a change from a guanine to citosine at nucleotide 238, which leads to a substitution of an alanine for a proline with a 100-fold reduction in enzyme activity. The TPMT*3A variant is the result of a change from a guanine to a adenine at nucleotide 460, which leads to a substitution of an alanine for a threonine at position 154; and the TPMT*3C variant is the result of a change from adenine to guanine at nucleotide 719, which leads to a substitution of a threonine for a cysteine at position 240, and this leads to severe toxicity of 6-MP and 6-TG due to reduced clearance of these drugs (Bertino, 2013).

Moreover, the balance between the nucleotide thioguanine 6- (6-TGN) in erythrocytes and methylated metabolite 6- (6-MMON) impacts the effectiveness of the treatment of ALL. Hepatotoxicity is a common complication associated with the use of 6-MP (Adam de Beaumais et al., 2011).

Individuals with nonfunctional TPMT alleles are at high risk of toxicity if treated with conventional doses of thiopurines (100% risk), and they also inactivate the active thiopurine drugs because they have no pathways of methylation. Patients who have one of two nonfunctional alleles are at high risk of hematological toxicity. Moreover, patients with high TPMT activity are at high risk of relapse when treated with a standard dose of 6-MP and must receive the full dose of thiopurine (Appell et al., 2013).

Genotypic testing can identify individuals with TPMT enzyme deficiency because the three alleles (TPMT *2A, TPMT *3A, TPMT *3C) account for 95% of individuals with reduced TPMT activity. It is also possible to perform phenotypic testing, with the identification of levels of thiopurine nucleotides or TPMT activity of erythrocytes. However, coadministration of drugs and blood transfusion may interfere with the results (U.S. Food and Drug Administration, 2011).

It is important to note that fatal toxicity has been observed even among patients with normal TPMT enzyme activity. The recommendation is that patients should be monitored for complete blood count and renal function, and normal TPMT enzyme activity should not eliminate clinical monitoring (Adam de Beaumais et al., 2011).

Pyrimidine Analogs

5-fluorouracil (5-FU) is a pyrimidine analog that is metabolized to 5-monophosphate that inhibits thymidylate syntase (TS). It is a drug used in a variety of solid tumors, among them gastrointestinal, breast, head, and neck tumors. The primary mechanism of cytotoxicity of 5-FU is the inhibition of the TS of the metabolite 5-fluoro-2'-deoxy-uridine-5'-monophosphate (5-FdUMP). 5-FU can be incorporated directly into RNA, interfering with RNA transcription; and, less frequently, in DNA, interfering with replication. One part of 5-FU exerts its cytotoxic effects because most is metabolized to inactive metabolites (Bertino, 2013).

Dihydropyrimidine dehydrogenase (DPD) is the first step in the catabolism of py-rimidines, including 5-FU and capecitabine. It is expressed in the liver and metabolizes more than 80% of the administered 5-FU, while the other 20% is excreted in the urine (Papanastasopoulos & Stebbing, 2014).

It is expected that 5% to 10% of the population has DPD deficiency activity. The DPYD gene (the gene coding for DPD) is complex, and several variants have been identified (Zdanowicz & American Society of Health-System Pharmacists, 2010). Although total deficiency is a rare event, reduced levels of enzyme activity are more common, especially in African Americans and women (Bertino, 2013). DPD deficiency is related to the development of severe toxicity manifested by diarrhea, mucositis, stomatitis, and neutropenia (Caudle et al., 2013).

The variant splice site IVS14+1 G> A results in a deficient DPD, leading to toxicity of 5-FU (Saif, 2013). Heterozygous patients with intermediate activity and who present a reduction in enzyme activity have the recommendation of a 50% reduction of the initial dose with toxicity evaluation. Homozygous patients or those with a deficiency in enzyme activity must have other drugs in their treatment plan (Caudle et al., 2013).

Manufacturers of 5-FU in different routes of administration did not recommend administration to individuals with DPD deficiency. However, the predictive value positive test for toxicity grade 3 or 4 is 46%; the reduced DPD activity was observed in patients with no mutation DPYD. At this time, testing for DPD deficiency is not recommended for commercial use (Amstutz, Froehlich, & Largiadèr, 2011).

Gemcitabine is used in various carcinomas: non-small cell lung cancer, pancreatic, bladder, and breast cancer. Gemcitabine is a prodrug and requires activation of cellular nucleoside transporters and intracellular phosphorylation. Inactivation of almost 90% of the administered dose is the metabolism of 2'-2'-difluorodeoxyuridina through actions of cytidine deaminase (CDA; Candelaria et al., 2010). It has a narrow therapeutic window, and its effects are well tolerated, with severe hematologic toxicity in 5% to 10% of cases (Zdanowicz & American Society of Health-System Pharmacists, 2010).

The G208A variant designated CDA*3, in which a threonine is replaced by alanine at amino acid 70, shows a decrease in the clearance of gemcitabine with increased incidence of neutropenia when coadministration of 5-FU occurs (Baker et al., 2013). However, no recommendation in clinical practice is observed.

Antimetabolites of Folic Acid

The antimetabolites of folic acid, which block dihydrofolate reductase (DHFR), have a broad tumor spectrum. The inhibition of the conversion of folic acid into tetrahydrofolate results in cell cycle arrest with inhibition of the synthesis of DNA, RNA, and protein. Thymidylate syntase (TS) variants have been suggested as involved in the efficacy of folic acid antimetabolites (Zdanowicz & American Society of Health-System Pharmacists, 2010).

Among the antimetabolites is methotrexate (MTX), which enters in the cell and is transported by reducing folate carrier (RFC), and its mechanism of action is inhibition of DHFR (Ongaro et al., 2009). There is evidence that MTX toxicity can be altered by single nucleotide polymorphisms (SNPs) in several genes involved in the folate pathway. The RFC1, MTHFR, and DHFR genes are associated with the occurrence of toxicity in the administration of MTX (Niedzielska, Węcławek-Tompol, Matkowska-Kocjan, & Chybicka, 2013).

Ongaro et al. (2009) evaluated 122 Italian adults with ALL and noted that MTHFR 677C>T was associated with liver toxicity, leukopenia, and gastrointestinal toxicity. The 677T allele exhibited a five- to six-fold increase in leukopenia and liver toxicity. The deletion of 19 base pairs at both DHFR alleles increased liver toxicity. Associations between these polymorphisms and survival were also observed (Ongaro et al., 2009).

TS variants are important in pharmcogenetic antimetabolites of folic acid. Drugs such as MTX inhibit this enzyme in the neoplastic cell to change cell metabolism. Changes in gene promoter may lead to a worse outcome in treatment with MTX, which may indicate the test for the individualization of treatment (Zdanowicz & American Society of Health-System Pharmacists, 2010).

Type 1 Topoisomerase Inhibitors

Irinotecan is a semisynthetic derivative of camptothecin, which has antineoplastic activity, due to inhibition of the enzyme topoisomerase type I, required for DNA replication (Zdanowicz & American Society of Health-System Pharmacists, 2010). It is used for treatment of metastatic colorectal cancer.

The biotransformation of irinotecan SN-38 by carboxylesterases is essential for the antitumor activity of irinotecan. SN-38 has an antitumor activity 1,000 times superior to irinotecan. Polymorphic variations in carboxylesterases may affect the efficacy of irinotecan. SN-38 is inactivated by UDP-glucoronosiltransferanse (UGT), including UGT1A1 and UGT1A7, which give rise to SN-38 glucoronides, which are eliminated via bile and urine. The UDP glucorosiltransferases are a family of enzymes responsible for the glucuronidation of drugs, steroids, bilirubin, and other soluble molecules to form molecules that can be secreted. Irinotecan has a narrow therapeutic window, with side effects such as myelosuppression (mainly leukopenia and thrombocytopenia) and diarrhea, which is seen in 29% to 44% of patients (de Jong, de Jonge, Verweij, & Mathijssen, 2006; Lankisch et al., 2008).

The adverse effects of irinotecan are associated with changes in the activity of UGT present in Gilbert's syndrome, characterized by a variant called UGT1A1*28, which has a TA repeat in the promoter region of the UGT1A1 gene (which has seven TAs repeats compared with six) with no apparent reduction in the excretion of hepatic expression. The reduction in the levels of UGT1A1 results in reduced excretion of SN-38 and hepatic toxicity due to high levels of SN-38. Patients with UGT1A1*28 variants have an increased risk of neutropenia, severe diarrhea, and death through the use of irinotecan (Lankisch et al., 2008). In the Lankisch et al. (2008) study, the UGT1A1/UGT1A7 haplotypes were able to predict the risk of adverse events. Lévesque et al. (2013), in a prospective study of 167 Italian patients, identified other SNPs in the gene UGT1A besides the UGT1A1*28 (such as UGT1A6, UGT1A7, UGT1A9) that are associated with irinotecan toxicity. Inoue et al. (2013) found that UGT1A1*6/*28, UGT1A7*3/*3, UGT1A9*1/*1 polymorphisms have been associated with increased toxicity using irinotecan in Japanese patients.

According to Hertz & McLeod (2013), there is a tolerance dose of irinotecan ranging from 130mg/m² to 390mg/m² depending on the genotype. In a meta-analysis it was observed that neutropenia is associated with irinotecan, dose-dependent on the genotype UGT1A1*28: Neutropenia was higher in the group receiving doses greater than 150mg/m² (Hoskins, Goldberg, Qu, Ibrahim, & McLeod, 2007). The greatest risk of severe diarrhea was also observed in women with the UGT1A1*28 genotype and those who received high doses of irinotecan (Hu, Yu, & Zhao, 2010).

In the United States, 10% of Caucasians are homozygous for UGT1A1*28, and 40% are heterozygous (de Jong et al., 2006).

Cost-effectiveness of pharmacogenomic testing has shown the usefulness of irinotecan in Caucasians, African Americans, and also in medium- and high-dose regimens, given that a relationship between the occurrence of effects and dose regimen used is observed (Bertino 2013). Although evidence of cost-effectiveness in some populations has been observed, the test does not have wide acceptance (Bertino, 2013).

It is important to note that the UGT1A1 polymorphisms and the presence of hyperbilirubinemia are also phenomenons observed in the use of nilotinib. According to Shibata et al. (2014), patients with the UGT1A1 genotype were poor metabolizers (UGT1A1*6/*6 or UGT1A1*6/*28) with severe toxicity.

Selective Estrogen Receptor Modulators (Tamoxifen and Raloxifen)

Tamoxifen (TMX) and raloxifen are selective estrogen receptor modulators (SERMs) and act as antagonists of estrogen in the estrogen receptor in breast tumors that are positive for these receptors. Many breast tumors express estrogen receptor alpha, which in the presence of estrogen, acts as a promoter of neoplastic growth. Inhibition of estrogen receptor reduces the proliferative activity in breast cancer cells. SERMs block estrogen's interaction with the receptor, thereby reducing cell proliferation (Zdanowicz & American Society of Health-System Pharmacists, 2010).

TMX is prescribed for the treatment of breast cancer in premenopausal women positive for breast cancer, and raloxifen may be prescribed for similar postmenopausal patients (Zdanowicz & American Society of Health-System Pharmacists, 2010).

TMX is metabolized to its active metabolite N-desmethyl and 4-TMX hydroxytamoxyfen, by several CYP450 enzymes, including CYP2D6, CYP3A4, CYP2C9, CYP2C19, and CYP2B6. Importantly, N-desmethyl TMX is metabolized by CYP2D6 to endoxifen. Endofixen is 30 to 100 times more potent than TMX in suppressing cellular estrogen and is considered responsible for the pharmacological effects of TMX (Fleeman et al., 2011).

The CYP2D6 gene is highly polymorphic, with more than 80 alleles having been identified. The activity of TMX is not only influenced by genetic factors but also by using drugs, such as selective serotonin reuptake inhibitors (SSRIs), which may affect the phenotype of patients (Fleeman et al., 2011). The CYP2D6*4 variant, present in 17% to 21% of Caucasians, has a change of G to A in the first base pair of exon 4, resulting in a splice site, and the generation of a stop codon. Individuals who are homozygous for CYP2D6*4 lack CYP2D6 activity, and heterozygous CYP2D6*4 are slow metabolizers. Thus, this group has a high risk of recurrence (Zdanowicz & American Society of Health-System Pharmacists, 2010).

In an analysis of three cohorts, Fleeman et al. (2011) found that extensive metabolizers and intermediate metabolizers had more hot flashes than poor metabolizers. According to the authors, from the analysis of 63 studies, it was not possible to say that the CYP2D6 test is clinically effective or cost-effective (Fleeman et al., 2011). To Kiyotani, Mushiroda, Nakamura, & Zembutsu (2012), the association between CYP2D6 genotype and results are still controversial.

Taxanes

Taxanes are agents that act in stabilizing microtubules and preventing depolymerization. Taxanes include paclitaxel, which is a derivative of dipertenas plane, and docetaxel and cabazitaxel, which are semisynthetic (Galsky, Dritselis, Kirkpatrick, & Oh, 2010). Taxanes are used for treatment of solid tumors, usually carcinomas, among them head and neck, breast, ovarian, and prostate (cabazitaxel).

Taxanes have a narrow therapeutic window with several adverse events, the most significant being hematological and neurological events. It is not clear which SNPs can guide treatment with taxanes because there is no consensus in the literature (Bergmann et al., 2011; Krens, McLeod, & Hertz, 2013). Among the candidate genes are CYP3A4/3A5, CYP2C8, ABCB1, CYP1B1, and b-tubilin (Krens et al., 2013).

There are reports that polymorphisms in TUBB2A gene encoding a b-tubulin isotype acts as a protective factor in the occurrence of peripheral neuropathy (Hertz, McLeod, & Hoskins, 2009).

Alkylating Agents

Cyclophosphamide is an alkylating agent widely used in the treatment of solid tumors as well as hematological tumors. It is a prodrug that depends on the bioactivation of 4-hydroxycyclophosphamide for its cytotoxic activity. Bioactivation is highly variable between individuals; CYP2B6, CYP2C19, and CYP3A4 genes were identified as associated with the metabolism of the agent (Zanger & Klein, 2013).

Cisplatin is used for a variety of solid tumors in adults and children. However, it has dose-limiting toxicities, such as ototoxicity, nephrotoxicity, and peripheral neuropathy.

Ototoxicity affects between 10% and 25% of adults and 25% to 90% of children. Variations in COMT, XPC, ABCC3, GST3, and LRP3 genes were associated with ototoxicity, but the clinical utility is uncertain, and it is necessary to validate the markers (Lee et al., 2014; Mukherjea & Rybak, 2011). For the TPMT gene, the U.S. Food and Drug Administration (FDA) included in the package insert a warning of the high risk of ototoxicity in patients with TPMT*3B and *3C (Lee et al., 2014).

Anthracycline Antibiotics

The anthracycline antibiotics have highly effective antitumor activity and are used in the treatment of various solid tumors in children and adults. Heart disease is the major dose-limiting toxicity (Blanco et al, 2012; Lee et al., 2014). The primary route of metabolism of anthracycline is the two-electron reduction at C-13 carbonyl group on the side of each anthracycline, resulting in the formation of metabolic alcoholics. The development of cardiomyopathy is related to the accumulation of metabolites. The variability in the formation of these metabolites may influence the risk of cardiomyopathy because the synthesis of metabolites is catalyzed by CBRs (carbonyl reductase myocardial citosalia), which is encoded by a gene on chromosome 21 (Blanco et al., 2012).

Several genes have been identified as potentially associated with cardiotoxicity of anthracyclines: SCL28A3, ABC, NADPH, CBR SULT2B1, GST, CAT, and UGT1A6. Replication studies show that SCL28A3 and UGT1A6 variants are markers that are associated with the risk, which makes them potential markers of cardiotoxicity (Lee et al., 2014).

Blanco et al. (2012) evaluated 317 survivors with childhood cancer and found that individuals homozygous for an allele in the gene *CBR23* contributed to risk, although risk was not dose-dependent. For individuals with allele A, no toxicity in low or moderate doses was observed, but at higher doses (> 250mg/m²), toxicity was observed regardless of the outcome (Blanco et al., 2012).

Somatic Variants: Selected Therapeutics

Cancer is a genomic disease. During the progression of cancer, genetic changes occur in subpopulations of cells, leading to disease development.

Somatic changes offer opportunities to identify markers for diagnosis, determine the prognosis, and make the choice of therapy. With the knowledge and understanding of tumor biology, it has been possible to develop drugs that have targeted specific genetic alterations along with the possibility to identify groups of patients who will respond to treatment and those who are at high risk for recurrence.

The amplification of the HER2 gene with protein overexpression occurs in approximately 15% of patients with breast cancer, and its presence is related to worse disease-free survival and overall survival. For patients with metastatic disease and HER2-positive tumors, four agents are approved: trastuzumab, lapatinib, pertuzumab, ado-trastuzumab emtansine (Figueroa-Magalhães, Jelovac, Connolly, & Wolff, 2014; Lamond & Younis, 2014). The use of trastuzumab was extended to patients with gastric adenocarcinoma showing overexpression of HER2 (Albarello, Pecciarini, & Doglioni, 2011).

The EGFR (epidermal growth factor receptor)—also known as HER1, or Erb—is a tyrosine kinase. It has functions in cellular differentiation and proliferation, and its activation occurs in solid tumors, such as non-small cell lung cancer (NSCLC), head/neck cancer (HSNCC), and colorectal cancer (CRC; Yokota, 2014).

Overexpression of EGFR has been observed in various tumors. In HSNCC, it is a prognostic marker and is an important therapeutic target (Yokota, 2014). In EGFR signaling are several genes, including K-RAS. K-RAS is mutated in 15% to 30% of lung tumors, 40% to 50% of CRC, and up to 90% of pancreatic tumors (Dempke & Heinemann, 2010).

For the selection of the treatment with EGFR inhibitors (EGFR-TKIs: geftinib, erlonitib) in patients with lung cancer, it has been found that the tumors with deletion of exon 19 L858R EGFR mutation showed increased sensitivity to treatment with tyrosine kinase inhibitors (Khozin et al., 2014; Okamoto, 2010). However, during treatment with EGFR-TKIs, the development of the phenomenon of resistance is observed. It has been shown that up to 70% of tumors that develop resistance to EGFR tyrosine kinase inhibitors present the mutation T790M and amplification of MET gene; therefore, these changes should be related to resistance to antineoplastic therapy (Okamoto, 2010).

In metastatic CRC, mutations in the K-RAS gene contraindicate cetuximab and panitumumab therapy. In a meta-analysis to verify pharmacogenomic benefit, Lin, Webber, Senger, Holmes, and Whitlock (2011) found that BRAF is a better predictor than K-RAS and also that the biomarker is associated with worsening in progression and survival. According to the authors, the other tests besides K-RAS are of limited use in clinical practice (Lin et al., 2011).

Among various biomarkers in CRC, TS has been extensively evaluated. TS is expressed in normal and neoplastic cells and is an enzyme that is essentially involved in the synthesis of thymidylate. Because TS is the target of 5-FU, its expression has been investigated. High TS expression is associated with poor response to 5-FU (Longley, Harkin, & Johnston, 2003).

Four new target drugs have revolutionized the treatment response of melanoma: ipilimumab, vemurafenib, dabrafenib, and trametinb (Olszanski, 2014). The latter three act in the MAPK signaling pathway. Vemurafenib and dabrafenib are BRAF inhibitors and are indicated for patients with BRAF V600E mutation (Flaherty, Yasothan, & Kirkpatrick, 2011). Vemurafenib represents an improvement in patient survival compared with the standard regimen (dacarbazine; Chapman et al., 2011). About 40% to 50% of melanomas have mutations in BRAF; and of those, 90% have the V600E mutation. Trametinib is also a therapeutic option that acts by inhibiting MEK (Olszanski, 2014). Ipilimimumab blocks cytotoxic T-lymphocytic antigin-4 (CTLA-4) but has not as yet shown an increase in the survival of melanoma patients, requiring the development of biomarkers to better select patients for response and toxicity (Sondak, Redman, DeVita, Hellman, & Rosenberg, 2005).

The reciprocal translocation t (9; 22) called the "Philadelphia chromosome" (Ph) results in the fusion of the BCR and ABL proteins, leading to formation of the protein tyrosine kinase BCR-ABL. This leads to a constitutive protein tyrosine kinase activity, and it is most frequently observed in chronic myeloid leukemia (CML) but can also occur in ALL.

Imatinib was the first inhibitor of tyrosine kinase BCR-ABL fusion approved for the treatment of CML (de Lavallade et al., 2008.) The drug binds to an inactive conformation of BCR-ABL protein and also binds PDGGFRA (derived growth factor alpha platelets) and protein kinase KIT (growth factor receptor of stem cells), which can be used in cancers that have alterations in these proteins.

Additionally, imatinib is used in GIST (gastrointestinal stromal sarcomas) that are c-kit–positive (Bertino, 2013). Mutations in c-kit are observed in more than 90% of cases, and patients with mutations in exon 11 are those with better response (Corless, Barnett, & Heinrich, 2011). A c-kit is a type of receptor tyrosine kinase and a type of tumor marker (NCI, 2014).

Treatment with imatinib aims at complete remission: cytogenetic and hematologic response. However, imatinib fails to eliminate the stem cells from bone marrow; therefore, some patients develop resistance to imatinib. The mechanisms of resistance are related to amplification and overexpression of mRNA and protein. However, the most common mechanism is the occurrence of mutations in the ABL gene. To overcome imatinib resistance, other drugs have been developed—among them, nilotinib, which is 30 times more potent than imatinib. Dasatinib has also been used; however, in addition to being a potent inhibitor of BCR-ABL activity, it is an inhibitor of Src family, KIT, and PDGFR (Breccia & Alimena, 2014; Shah et al., 2014).

After the approval of nilotinib and dasatinib, bosutinib and ponatinib—indicated for CML and exhibit progression or resistance to previous treatment—were developed. These drugs are indicated for patients with CML with T315I mutation and have a substantial response rate in this group of patients (Bose Park, Al-Khafaji, & Grant, 2013).

The molecular target drugs are a trend in oncology, and they are associated with conventional drugs. There is an increasing investment in the development of these drugs as well as their markers for the selection of patients who may be more responsive to treatment.

Table 8.1 shows drugs in oncology that have biomarkers identified by the FDA and evidence in the literature for its application.

Table 8.1   Pharmacogenomic Biomarkers in Oncology Drugs

Drug	Gene Nomenclature*	Main Indication	Pharmacogenomic Biomarker/ Recommendation
Afatinib	EGFR	Metastatic NSCLC	Afatinib should be used only in tumors with EGFR deletions in exon 19 or exon 21 detected by an FDA-approved test (Mancheril, Aubrey Waddell, & Solimando, 2014; Wu et al., 2014).
Anastrozole	ESR1, PGR	Postmenopausal breast cancer hormonal receptor-positive	The status of the hormonal receptor should be tested prior to therapy given that anastrozole is not effective in tumors that are hormonal receptor-negative.
Arsenic trioxide	PML/RARA	Promyelocytic leukemia	Arsenic trioxide should be used only in the presence of t(15;17) or PML/RAR alpha (Lo-Coco et al., 2013).
Bosutinib	BCR/ABL1	CML: with resistance or intolerance to anterior treatment	Bosutinib is indicated only in patients with CML Philadelphia chromosome–positive (Ph+), also seen in ALL. The drug is metabolized by CYP3A; therefore, the concomitant use of CYP3A inhibitors and inductors should be avoided (Caudle et al., 2013; Hanaizi et al., 2014).

Drug	Gene Nomenclature*	Main Indication	Pharmacogenomic Biomarker/ Recommendation
Busulfan	Ph+ Chromosome	CML	Philadelphia Chromosome Positive (Ph+) should be detected by an FDA-approved test.
Capecitabine	DPYD	CRC: adjuvant therapy and also metastatic disease; Breast cancer: metastatic disease	The drug is contraindicated in patients with DPD deficiency. Severe toxicity (stomatitis, diarrhea, neutropenia, and neurotoxicity) is observed (Amstutz et al., 2011; Caudle et al., 2013). There are drug-drug interactions caused by CYP2C9 interference. CYP2C9 subtracts should be used carefully.
Cetuximab	EGFR	HSNCC: local and advanced; Metastatic CRC	In CRC, EGFR status should be determined. The drug is not effective in tumors with somatic mutations in K-RAS in codons 12 e 13 (exon 2); therefore, K-RAS status should be determined prior cetuximab administration (Dempke & Heinemann, 2010; Karapetis et al., 2008). In HSNCC, because almost all tumors express EGFR, it is not necessary to verify its expression (Yokota, 2014).

continues

Table 8.1   Pharmacogenomic Biomarkers in Oncology Drugs   *(continued)*

Drug	Gene Nomenclature*	Main Indication	Pharmacogenomic Biomarker/ Recommendation
Cisplatin	TPMT	Variety of solid tumors in adults and children	The *TPMT**3B and TPMT*3C are associated with an increased risk of ototoxicity in children who received conventional doses of cisplatin. Although the association is high, there is no recommendation of genetic testing. One-half of children without these genotypes will develop severe ototoxicity. The FDA recommends audiometric testing at baseline, during treatment, and afterward (Brock et al., 2012; Pussegoda et al., 2013; Wang & Weinshilboum, 2006).
Crizotinib	ALK	Metastatic NSCLC	Crizotinib should be used only in tumors that are anaplastic lymphoma kinase (ALK)– positive as detected by an FDA-approved test (Camidge et al., 2012; Shaw et al., 2013).

The drug is metabolized by CYP3A; therefore, drugs that are inducers or inhibitors of CYP3A should be administered with caution and analyzed carefully or avoided. |

Drug	Gene Nomenclature*	Main Indication	Pharmacogenomic Biomarker/ Recommendation
Dabrafenib	BRAF G6PD	Unresectable or metastatic melanoma	Should be prescribed for melanoma whose tumors present BRAF V600E mutation detected by an FDA-approved test (Hauschild et al., 2012; Olszanski, 2014). Patients with G6PD (glucose-6-phosphate dehydrogenase deficiency) should be monitored for signs of hemolytic anemia because G6PD confers a potential risk. Avoid concurrent administration of strong inducers or inducers of CYP3A4 or CYP2C8. Concurrent use with agents that synthetize with CYP3A4, CYP2C8, CYP2C9, CYP2C19, or CYP2B6 may result in loss of efficacy of these agents.

continues

Table 8.1 Pharmacogenomic Biomarkers in Oncology Drugs *(continued)*

Drug	Gene Nomenclature*	Main Indication	Pharmacogenic Biomarker/ Recommendation
Ibritumomab tiuxetan	MS4A1	Relapsed or refractory, low-grade or follicular B-cell non-Hodgkin's lymphoma (NHL)	The status of CD-20 receptor on B-cell non-Hodgkin's lymphomas (NHL) should be evaluated prior to therapy (Bodet-Milin et al., 2013).
Imatinib	KIT BCR/ABL1 PDGFRB FIP1L1/PDGFRA	Ph+ CML Ph+ ALL Adult patients with myelodysplastic/ myeloproliferative diseases (MDS/MPD) associated with platelet-derived growth factor receptor (PDGFR) gene rearrangements Patients with KIT (CD117)–positive unresectable and/or metastatic GIST	Ph+ status should be determined in CML and ALL (Bansal, 2014). The presence of *KIT* mutation should be confirmed prior to Imatinib administration in GISTs (Zhi, Zhou, Wang, & Xu, 2013).

Drug	Gene Nomenclature*	Main Indication	Pharmacogenic Biomarker/ Recommendation
Irinotecan	UGT1A1	Metastatic CRC	Individuals who are homozygous for the UGT1A1*28 allele are at increased risk for neutropenia following initiation of irinotecan treatment (Lankisch et al., 2008). A reduction in the starting dose should be considered for patients known to be homozygous for the UGT1A1*28 allele (de Jong et al., 2006).
Lapatinib	ERBB2	Advanced or metastatic breast cancer whose tumors overexpress HER2	For patients with breast cancer, the status of hormonal receptor (positive) and also the presence of HER2 amplification should be evaluated prior to therapy (Figueroa-Magalhães et al., 2014; Yan, Parker, Schwab, & Kurzrock, 2014).
Letrozole	ESR1, PGR	Breast cancer hormonal receptor-positive	For patients with breast cancer, the status of hormonal receptor (positive) should be evaluated prior to therapy (Goss et al., 2005).
Mercaptopurine	TPMT	ALL	Homozygous-deficient patients (two nonfunctional alleles), if given usual doses of 6-MP, accumulate excessive concentrations of active thioguanine nucleotides, predisposing them to toxicity (Appell et al., 2013).

continues

Table 8.1 Pharmacogenomic Biomarkers in Oncology Drugs *(continued)*

Drug	Gene Nomenclature*	Main Indication	Pharmacogenic Biomarker/ Recommendation
Nilotinib	BCR/ABL1	CML Ph+	Ph+ status should be determined in CML (Breccia & Alimena, 2014). UGT1A1*28 has been linked to an increased risk of hyperbilirubinemia in patients with CML who receive nilotinib (Shibata et al., 2014). Avoid concomitant use of strong inhibitors or inducers of CYP3A4.
Obinutuzumab	MS4A1	Chronic lymphocytic leukemia (CLL)	The status of CD-20 receptor on CLL cell should be evaluated prior to therapy (Rai & Barrientos, 2014).
Omacetaxine	BCR/ABL	Chronic or accelerated phase CML	Omacetaxine has improved actived T315I mutated Bcr-Abl CML (Bose et al., 2013).
Panitumumab	EGFR KRAS	Metastatic CRC	Panitumad should be used only in wild-type tumors; therefore, K-RAS mutational status by an FDA-approved test should be performed prior to administration.
Pazopanib	UGT1A1	Advanced RCC Advanced soft tissue sarcoma (STS)	The genotype UGT1A1*28/*28 can lead to hyperbilirubinemia during pazopanib treatment (Xu et al., 2010). Avoid co-administration with inducers or inhibitors of CYP3A4.

Drug	Gene Nomenclature*	Main Indication	Pharmacogenic Biomarker/ Recommendation
Pertuzumab	ERBB2	Breast cancer HER2-positive	Determination of HER2 overexpression should be performed by laboratories using an FDA-approved test (Lamond & Younis, 2014).
Ponatinib	BCR –ABL T315I	T315I-positive CML or T315Ipositive ALL Ph+	Presence of T315I mutation should be determined prior use of therapy (Bose et al., 2013). Avoid co-administration with inducers or inhibitors of CYP3A4.
Rituximab	MS4A1	B-cell NHL	The status of CD-20 receptor on B-cell NHL should be evaluated prior to therapy.
Tamoxifen	ESR1, PGR F5, F2	Breast cancer or breast cancer prevention	The status of hormonal receptor should be evaluated prior to therapy.
Tositumomab	MS4A1	B-cell NHL	The status of CD-20 receptor on B-cell NHL should be evaluated prior use of therapy (Srinivasan & Mukherji, 2011).
Thioguanine	TPMT	ALL	Homozygous-deficient patients (two nonfunctional alleles), if given usual doses of thioguanine, accumulate cellular concentrations of active thioguanine nucleotides, predisposing them to 6-TG toxicity.

continues

Table 8.1   Pharmacogenomic Biomarkers in Oncology Drugs   *(continued)*

Drug	Gene Nomenclature*	Main Indication	Pharmacogenic Biomarker/Recommendation
Trametinib	BRAF	Malignant melanoma	Status of *BRAF V600E* or V600K mutation should be performed by laboratories using FDA-approved tests (Luke & Hodi, 2013).
Trastuzumab	ERBB2	Breast cancer HER2-positive Gastric cancer HER2-positive	Determination of HER2 overexpression should be performed by laboratories using FDA-approved tests (Figueroa-Magalhães et al., 2014).
Vemurafenib	BRAF	Malignant melanoma	Status of *BRAF V600E* mutation should be performed by laboratories using FDA-approved tests (Luke & Hodi, 2013).

* Gene names according to HGNC HUGO Gene Nomenclature (http://www.genenames.org)

Source: U.S. Department of Heath & Human Services, U.S. Food and Drug Administration (http://www.fda.gov/drugs/scienceresearch/researchareas/pharmacogenetics/ucm083378.htm).

Nursing and Ethical Considerations

Given that SNPs are specific in subpopulations, the research of ancestry during interview can help health professionals during data interpretation. This further reinforces the need for accurate patient histories.

Although more than 20 chemotherapeutic agents have pharmacogenetic markers on the FDA list, there is a clear disconnect between the markers and the dose recommendations. Only 6-MP, 6-TG, nilotinib, and irinotecan have recommendations for dose modifications based on genomic profile.

In certain individuals, abnormal drug responses may be due to pharmacokinetic or pharmacodynamic responses resulting from SNPs. The main source of pharmacokinetic variability is due to genetic polymorphism of enzymes, especially cytochrome P450 System, CYP450 (Cooper et al., 2005), whereas a significant proportion of drugs used in cancer treatment are substrates of the isoenzyme CYP450 (see Table 8.1) and the target of drug-drug interaction (DDI). The occurrence of this event can lead to therapeutic failure or increased toxicity. Oncologic nurses should be aware of the vulnerable groups of patients, such as those undergoing *polypharmacy* (use of five or more medications), elderly patients, those with presence of comorbidities, or/and those with hepatic or renal dysfunction (Chen & Cheung, 2014). For more on polypharmacy, see Chapter 7.

Ethical aspects related to pharmacogenomics, which can lead to inequalities in the health system, should be considered, especially in the poorest countries. Costs relating to the development, manufacturing, and obtaining approval for genetic testing are extremely high. Moreover, ethnic genetic differences are not always covered, and thus many patients from less-affluent scenarios would be excluded from the benefits of advances in genomics technologies (Carr, Alfirevic, & Pirmohamed, 2014).

Questions

Individuals with nonfunctional TPMT alleles are at high risk of toxicity if treated with conventional doses of:

   a.   Oymirimidines, such as 5-FU and capecitabina

   b.   Thiopurines, such as 6-MP and 6-TG *

   c.   Topoisomerase inhibitors, such as irinotecan and topotecan

   d.   Taxanes, such as paclitaxel and docetaxel

In metastatic colorectal cancer prior use of cetuximab, which phamacogenomic test should be performed?

   a.   HER2 protein overexpression

   b.   c-kit mutation

   c.   K-RAS wild-type status *

   d.   TS expression status

What are the factors that justify the use of strategies in pharmacogenomics in cancer care?

   •   Anticancer drugs have therapeutic window. Variation in response between individuals is observed, and there are few methods available to monitor safety and effectiveness.

Key Points

Strategies in pharmacogenomics are relevant because the drugs have a narrow therapeutic window, there is a high degree of interindividual variability in the response, and there are few methods with which to monitor safety or effectiveness (Bertino, 2013).

In recent decades, with greater understanding of cancer biology, the development of targeted drugs has been one of the most used therapeutic strategies in cancer treatment. This reinforces the need for integrating concepts of molecular biology and genetics to nursing practice in the care of these patients.

Besides drug screening, pharmacogenomics has a potential role in identifying adverse events and can be used to help improve the quality of life of cancer patients. Selection of an appropriate therapy, early detection of complications, and appropriate intervention can reduce the suffering of patients during treatment arising from cancer therapy.

We observed that the clinical applicability of pharmacogenomic testing is still debatable in some cases because there is a need for the validation of data after the identification of markers in the research setting. Thus, nurses must recognize the limitations and discuss them with their clients. The discussion of the limitations of pharmacogenomic testing is crucial for the client to make an informed decision about the course of treatment.

References

Adam de Beaumais, T., Fakhoury, M., Medard, Y., Azougagh, S., Zhang, D., Yakouben, K., & Jacqz-Aigrain, E. (2011). Determinants of mercaptopurine toxicity in paediatric acute lymphoblastic leukemia maintenance therapy. *British Journal of Clinical Pharmacology, 71*(4), 575–584. doi: 10.1111/j.1365-2125.2010.03867.x

Albarello, L., Pecciarini, L., & Doglioni, C. (2011). HER2 testing in gastric cancer. *Advances in Anatomic Pathology, 18*(1), 53–59. doi: 10.1097/PAP.0b013e3182026d72

Amstutz, U., Froehlich, T. K., & Largiadèr, C. R. (2011). Dihydropyrimidine dehydrogenase gene as a major predictor of severe 5-fluorouracil toxicity. *Pharmacogenomics, 12*(9), 1321–1336. doi: 10.2217/pgs.11.72

Appell, M. L., Berg, J., Duley, J., Evans, W. E., Kennedy, M. A., Lennard, L., & Coulthard, S. A. (2013). Nomenclature for alleles of the thiopurine methyltransferase gene. *Pharmacogenetic Genomics, 23*(4), 242–248. doi: 10.1097/FPC.0b013e32835f1cc0

Baker, J. A., Wickremsinhe, E. R., Li, C. H., Oluyedun, O. A., Dantzig, A. H., Hall, S. D., & Guo, Y. (2013). Pharmacogenomics of gemcitabine metabolism: Functional analysis of genetic variants in cytidine deaminase and deoxycytidine kinase. *Drug Metabolism and Disposition, 41*(3), 541–545. doi: 10.1124/dmd.112.048769

Bansal, S. (2014). Is imatinib still the best choice as first-line oral TKI. *South Asian Journal of Cancer, 3*(1), 83–86. doi: 10.4103/2278-330X.126553

Bergmann, T. K., Gréen, H., Brasch-Andersen, C., Mirza, M. R., Herrstedt, J., Hølund, B., & Peterson, C. (2011). Retrospective study of the impact of pharmacogenetic variants on paclitaxel toxicity and survival in patients with ovarian cancer. *European Journal of Clinical Pharmacology, 67*(7), 693–700. doi: 10.1007/s00228-011-1007-6

Bertino, J. S. (2013). *Pharmacogenomics: An introduction and clinical perspective.* New York, NY: McGraw-Hill.

Blanco, J. G., Sun, C. L., Landier, W., Chen, L., Esparza-Duran, D., Leisenring, W., & Bhatia, S. (2012). Anthracycline-related cardiomyopathy after childhood cancer: role of polymorphisms in carbonyl reductase genes—a report from the Children's Oncology Group. *Journal of Clinical Oncology, 30*(13), 1415–1421. doi: 10.1200/JCO.2011.34.8987

Bodet-Milin, C., Ferrer, L., Pallardy, A., Eugène, T., Rauscher, A., Faivre-Chauvet, A., . . . Kraeber-Bodéré, F. (2013). Radioimmunotherapy of B-Cell Non-Hodgkin's Lymphoma. *Frontiers in Oncology, 3*, 177. doi: 10.3389/fonc.2013.00177

Bose, P., Park, H., Al-Khafaji, J., & Grant, S. (2013). Strategies to circumvent the T315I gatekeeper mutation in the Bcr-Abl tyrosine kinase. *Leukeumia Research Reports, 2*(1), 18–20. doi: 10.1016/j.lrr.2013.02.001

Breccia, M., & Alimena, G. (2014). Second-generation tyrosine kinase inhibitors (TKI) as salvage therapy for resistant or intolerant patients to prior TKIs. *Mediterrean Journal of Hematology and Infectious Diseases, 6*(1), e2014003. doi: 10.4084/MJHID.2014.003

Brock, P. R., Knight, K. R., Freyer, D. R., Campbell, K. C., Steyger, P. S., Blakley, B. W., & Neuwelt, E. A. (2012). Platinum-induced ototoxicity in children: A consensus review on mechanisms, predisposition, and protection, including a new International Society of Pediatric Oncology Boston ototoxicity scale. *Journal of Clinical Oncology, 30*(19), 2408–2417. doi: 10.1200/JCO.2011.39.1110

Carr, D. F., Alfirevic, A., & Pirmohamed, M. (2014). Pharmacogenomics: Current state-of-the-art. *Genes, 5*, 430–443; doi:10.3390/genes5020430

Camidge, D. R., Bang, Y. J., Kwak, E. L., Iafrate, A. J., Varella-Garcia, M., Fox, S. B., & Shaw, A. T. (2012). Activity and safety of crizotinib in patients with ALK-positive non-small-cell lung cancer: updated results from a phase 1 study. *The Lancet Oncology, 13*(10), 1011–1019. doi: 10.1016/S1470-2045(12)70344-3

Candelaria, M., de la Cruz-Hernández, E., Pérez-Cárdenas, E., Trejo-Becerril, C., Gutiérrez-Hernández, O., & Dueñas-González, A. (2010). Pharmacogenetics and pharmacoepigenetics of gemcitabine. *Medical Oncology, 27*(4), 1133–1143. doi: 10.1007/s12032-009-9349-y

Caudle, K. E., Thorn, C. F., Klein, T. E., Swen, J. J., McLeod, H. L., Diasio, R. B., & Schwab, M. (2013). Clinical Pharmacogenetics Implementation Consortium guidelines for dihydropyrimidine dehydrogenase genotype and fluoropyrimidine dosing. *Clinical Pharmacology & Therapeutics, 94*(6), 640–645. doi: 10.1038/clpt.2013.172

Chapman, P. B., Hauschild, A., Robert, C., Haanen, J. B., Ascierto, P., Larkin, J., . . . BRIM-3 Study Group. (2011). Improved survival with vemurafenib in melanoma with BRAF V600E mutation. *New England Journal of Medicine, 364*(26), 2507–2516. doi: 10.1056/NEJMoa1103782

Chen, L., & Cheung, W. Y. (2014). Potential drug interactions in patients with a history of cancer. *Current Oncology, 21*(2), e212–20. doi: 10.3747/co.21.1657.

Corless, C. L., Barnett, C. M., & Heinrich, M. C. (2011). Gastrointestinal stromal tumours: Origin and molecular oncology. *Nature Reviews Cancer, 11*(12), 865–878. doi: 10.1038/nrc3143

Cooper, R. S., Wolf-Maier, K., Luke, A., Adeyemo, A., Banegas, J. R., Forrester, T., . . . Thamm, M. (2005). An international comparative study of blood pressure in populations of European vs. African descent. *BMC Medicine, 3*(1), 2. doi:10.1186/1741-7015-3-2

Crona, D., & Innocenti, F. (2012). Can knowledge of germline markers of toxicity optimize dosing and efficacy of cancer therapy? *Biomarkers in Medicine, 6*(3), 349–362. doi: 10.2217/bmm.12.19

de Jong, F. A., de Jonge, M. J., Verweij, J., & Mathijssen, R. H. (2006). Role of pharmacogenetics in irinotecan therapy. *Cancer Letters, 234*(1), 90–106. doi: 10.1016/j.canlet.2005.04.040

de Lavallade, H., Apperley, J. F., Khorashad, J. S., Milojkovic, D., Reid, A. G., Bua, M., & Marin, D. (2008). Imatinib for newly diagnosed patients with chronic myeloid leukemia: Incidence of sustained responses in an intention-to-treat analysis. *Journal of Clinical Oncology, 26*(20), 3358–3363. doi: 10.1200/JCO.2007.15.8154

Dempke, W. C., & Heinemann, V. (2010). Ras mutational status is a biomarker for resistance to EGFR inhibitors in colorectal carcinoma. *Anticancer Research, 30*(11), 4673–4677.

Figueroa-Magalhães, M. C., Jelovac, D., Connolly, R. M., & Wolff, A. C. (2014). Treatment of HER2-positive breast cancer. *Breast, 23*(2), 128–136. doi: 10.1016/j.breast.2013.11.011

Flaherty, K. T., Yasothan, U., & Kirkpatrick, P. (2011). Vemurafenib. *Nature Reviews Drug Discovery, 10*(11), 811–812. doi: 10.1038/nrd3579

Fleeman, N., Martin Saborido, C., Payne, K., Boland, A., Dickson, R., Dundar, Y., & Walley, T. (2011). The clinical effectiveness and cost-effectiveness of genotyping for CYP2D6 for the management of women with breast cancer treated with tamoxifen: a systematic review. *Health Technology Assessment, 15*(33), 1–102. doi: 10.3310/hta15330

Galsky, M. D., Dritselis, A., Kirkpatrick, P., & Oh, W. K. (2010). Cabazitaxel. *Nature Reviews Drug Discovery, 9*(9), 677–678. doi: 10.1038/nrd3254

Goss, P. E., Ingle, J. N., Martino, S., Robert, N. J., Muss, H. B., Piccart, M. J., & Pater, J. L. (2005). Randomized trial of letrozole following tamoxifen as extended adjuvant therapy in receptor-positive breast cancer: Updated findings from NCIC CTG MA.17. *Journal of the National Cancer Institute, 97*(17), 1262–1271. doi: 10.1093/jnci/dji250

Hall, M. J., Reid, J. E., Burbidge, L. A., Pruss, D., Deffenbaugh, A. M., Frye, C., . . . Noll, W. W. (2009). BRCA1 and BRCA2 mutations in women of different ethnicities undergoing testing for hereditary breast-ovarian cancer. *Cancer, 115*(10), 2222–2233.

Hanaizi, Z., Unkrig, C., Enzmann, H., Camarero, J., Sancho-Lopez, A., Salmonson, T., & Pignatti, F. (2014). The European medicines agency review of bosutinib for the treatment of adult patients with chronic myelogenous leukemia: Summary of the scientific assessment of the committee for medicinal products for human use. *Oncologist, 19*(4), 421–425. doi: 10.1634/theoncologist.2013-0294

Hauschild, A., Grob, J. J., Demidov, L. V., Jouary, T., Gutzmer, R., Millward, M., & Chapman, P. B. (2012). Dabrafenib in BRAF-mutated metastatic melanoma: A multicentre, open-label, phase 3 randomised controlled trial. *Lancet, 380*(9839), 358–365. doi: 10.1016/S0140-6736(12)60868-X

Hertz, D. L., & McLeod, H. L. (2013). Use of pharmacogenetics for predicting cancer prognosis and treatment exposure, response and toxicity. *Journal of Human Genetics, 58*(6), 346–352. doi: 10.1038/jhg.2013.42

Hertz, D. L., McLeod, H. L., & Hoskins, J. M. (2009). Pharmacogenetics of breast cancer therapies. *Breast, 18*(Suppl 3), S59–63. doi: 10.1016/S0960-9776(09)70275-9

Hoskins, J. M., Goldberg, R. M., Qu, P., Ibrahim, J. G., & McLeod, H. L. (2007). UGT1A1*28 genotype and irinotecan-induced neutropenia: Dose matters. *Journal of the National Cancer Institute, 99*(17), 1290–1295. doi: 10.1093/jnci/djm115

Hu, Z. Y., Yu, Q., & Zhao, Y. S. (2010). Dose-dependent association between UGT1A1*28 polymorphism and irinotecan-induced diarrhoea: A meta-analysis. *European Journal of Cancer, 46*(10), 1856–1865. doi: 10.1016/j.ejca.2010.02.049

Inoue, K., Sonobe, M., Kawamura, Y., Etoh, T., Takagi, M., Matsumura, T., & Itoh, K. (2013). Polymorphisms of the UDP-glucuronosyl transferase 1A genes are associated with adverse events in cancer patients receiving irinotecan-based chemotherapy. *The Tohoku Journal of Experimental Medicine, 229*(2), 107–114.

Karapetis, C. S., Khambata-Ford, S., Jonker, D. J., O'Callaghan, C. J., Tu, D., Tebbutt, N. C., & Zalcberg, J. R. (2008). K-ras mutations and benefit from cetuximab in advanced colorectal cancer. *New England Journal of Medicine, 359*(17), 1757–1765. doi: 10.1056/NEJMoa0804385

Khozin, S., Blumenthal, G. M., Jiang, X., He, K., Boyd, K., Murgo, A., & Pazdur, R. (2014, July 1). U.S. Food and Drug Administration approval summary: Erlotinib for the first-line treatment of metastatic non-small cell lung cancer with epidermal growth factor receptor exon 19 deletions or exon 21 (L858R) substitution mutations. *Oncologist,* 774–779. doi: 10.1634/theoncologist.2014-0089

Kiyotani, K., Mushiroda, T., Nakamura, Y., & Zembutsu, H. (2012). Pharmacogenomics of tamoxifen: Roles of drug metabolizing enzymes and transporters. *Drug Metabolism and Pharmacokinetics, 27*(1), 122–131.

Krens, S. D., McLeod, H. L., & Hertz, D. L. (2013). Pharmacogenetics, enzyme probes and therapeutic drug monitoring as potential tools for individualizing taxane therapy. *Pharmacogenomics, 14*(5), 555–574. doi: 10.2217/pgs.13.33

Lamond, N. W., & Younis, T. (2014). Pertuzumab in human epidermal growth-factor receptor 2-positive breast cancer: Clinical and economic considerations. *International Journal of Women's Health, 6,* 509–521. doi: 10.2147/IJWH.S47357

Lankisch, T. O., Schulz, C., Zwingers, T., Erichsen, T. J., Manns, M. P., Heinemann, V., & Strassburg, C. P. (2008). Gilbert's syndrome and irinotecan toxicity: Combination with UDP-glucuronosyltransferase 1A7 variants increases risk. *Cancer Epidemiology, Biomarkers & Prevention, 17*(3), 695–701. doi: 10.1158/1055-9965.EPI-07-2517

Lee, J. W., Aminkeng, F., Bhavsar, A. P., Shaw, K., Carleton, B. C., Hayden, M. R., & Ross, C. J. (2014). The emerging era of pharmacogenomics: Current successes, future potential, and challenges. *Clinical Genetics, 86*(1), 21–28. doi: 10.1111/cge.12392

Lévesque, E., Bélanger, A. S., Harvey, M., Couture, F., Jonker, D., Innocenti, F., & Guillemette, C. (2013). Refining the UGT1A haplotype associated with irinotecan-induced hematological toxicity in metastatic colorectal cancer patients treated with 5-fluorouracil/irinotecan-based regimens. *Journal of Pharmacology and Experimental Therapeutics, 345*(1), 95–101. doi: 10.1124/jpet.112.202242

Lin, J. S., Webber, E. M., Senger, C. A., Holmes, R. S., & Whitlock, E. P. (2011). Systematic review of pharmacogenetic testing for predicting clinical benefit to anti-EGFR therapy in metastatic colorectal cancer. *American Journal of Cancer Research, 1*(5), 650–662.

Lo-Coco, F., Avvisati, G., Vignetti, M., Thiede, C., Orlando, S. M., Iacobelli, S., & Study Alliance Leukemia (2013). Retinoic acid and arsenic trioxide for acute promyelocytic leukemia. *New England Journal of Medicine, 369*(2), 111–121. doi: 10.1056/NEJMoa1300874

Longley, D. B., Harkin, D. P., & Johnston, P. G. (2003). 5-fluorouracil: Mechanisms of action and clinical strategies. *Nature Reviews Cancer, 3*(5), 330–338. doi: 10.1038/nrc1074

Luke, J. J., & Hodi, F. S. (2013). Ipilimumab, vemurafenib, dabrafenib, and trametinib: Synergistic competitors in the clinical management of BRAF mutant malignant melanoma. *Oncologist, 18*(6), 717–725. doi: 10.1634/theoncologist.2012-0391

Mancheril, B. G., Aubrey Waddell, J., & Solimando, D. A. (2014). Drug monographs: Afatinib and obinutuzumab. *Hospital Pharmacy, 49*(3), 237–241. doi: 10.1310/hpj4903-237

Mukherjea, D., & Rybak, L. P. (2011). Pharmacogenomics of cisplatin-induced ototoxicity. *Pharmacogenomics, 12*(7), 1039–1050. doi: 10.2217/pgs.11.48

National Cancer Institute. NCI Dictionary of Cancer Terms. C-kit. Retrieved from http://www.cancer.gov/dictionary?CdrID=44329

Niedzielska, E., Węcławek-Tompol, J., Matkowska-Kocjan, A., & Chybicka, A. (2013). The influence of genetic RFC1, MS and MTHFR polymorphisms on the risk of acute lymphoblastic leukemia relapse in children and the adverse effects of methotrexate. *Advances in Clinical and Experimental Medicine, 22*(4), 579–584.

O'Donnell, P. H., & Ratain, M. J. (2012). Germline pharmacogenomics in oncology: Decoding the patient for targeting therapy. *Molecular Oncology, 6*(2), 251–259. doi: 10.1016/j.molonc.2012.01.005

Okamoto, I. (2010). Epidermal growth factor receptor in relation to tumor development: EGFR-targeted anticancer therapy. *FEBS Journal, 277*(2), 309–315. doi: 10.1111/j.1742-4658.2009.07449.x

Olszanski, A. J. (2014). Current and future roles of targeted therapy and immunotherapy in advanced melanoma. *Journal of Managed Care Pharmacy, 20*(4), 346–356.

Ongaro, A., De Mattei, M., Della Porta, M. G., Rigolin, G., Ambrosio, C., Di Raimondo, F., & Gemmati, D. (2009). Gene polymorphisms in folate metabolizing enzymes in adult acute lymphoblastic leukemia: Effects on methotrexate-related toxicity and survival. *Haematologica, 94*(10), 1391–1398. doi: 10.3324/haematol.2009.008326

Papanastasopoulos, P., & Stebbing, J. (2014). Molecular basis of 5-fluorouracil-related toxicity: Lessons from clinical practice. *Anticancer Research, 34*(4), 1531–1535.

Pussegoda, K., Ross, C. J., Visscher, H., Yazdanpanah, M., Brooks, B., Rassekh, S. R., . . . CPNDS Consortium. (2013). Replication of TPMT and ABCC3 genetic variants highly associated with cisplatin-induced hearing loss in children. *Clinical Pharmacology & Therapeutics, 94*(2), 243–251. doi: 10.1038/clpt.2013.80

Rai, K. R., & Barrientos, J. C. (2014). Movement toward optimization of CLL therapy. *New England Journal of Medicine, 370*(12), 1160–1162. doi: 10.1056/NEJMe1400599

Saif, M. W. (2013). Dihydropyrimidine dehydrogenase gene (DPYD) polymorphism among Caucasian and non-Caucasian patients with 5-FU- and capecitabine-related toxicity using full sequencing of DPYD. *Cancer Genomics Proteomics, 10*(2), 89–92.

Shah, N. P., Guilhot, F., Cortes, J. E., Schiffer, C. A., le Coutre, P., Brümmendorf, T. H., & Saglio, G. (2014). Long-term outcome with dasatinib after imatinib failure in chronic-phase chronic myeloid leukemia: Follow-up of a phase 3 study. *Blood, 123*(15), 2317–2324. doi: 10.1182/blood-2013-10-532341

Shaw, A. T., Kim, D. W., Nakagawa, K., Seto, T., Crinó, L., Ahn, M. J., & Jänne, P. A. (2013). Crizotinib versus chemotherapy in advanced ALK-positive lung cancer. *New England Journal of Medicine, 368*(25), 2385–2394. doi: 10.1056/NEJMoa1214886

Shibata, T., Minami, Y., Mitsuma, A., Morita, S., Inada-Inoue, M., Oguri, T., & Ando, Y. (2014). Association between severe toxicity of nilotinib and UGT1A1 polymorphisms in Japanese patients with chronic myelogenous leukemia. *International Journal of Clinical Oncology, 19*(2), 391–396. doi: 10.1007/s10147-013-0562-5

Sondak, V. K., & Redman, B. G. (2005). Pharmacology of Cancer Biotherapeutics: Section 1: Interferons. In V. T. De Vita, S. Hellman, & S. A. Rosenberg (eds.), *Cancer, principles, and practice of oncology* (7th ed). Philadelphia: J. B. Lippincot.

Srinivasan, A., & Mukherji, S. K. (2011). Tositumomab and iodine I 131 tositumomab (Bexaar). *American Journal of Neuroradiology, 32*(4), 637–638. doi: 10.3174/ajnr.A2593

U.S. Food and Drug Administration (2011). Purinethol (mercaptopurine) 50mg Scored Tables. Retrieved from http://www.accessdata.fda.gov/drugsatfda_docs/label/2011/009053s032lbl.pdf

Wang, L., & Weinshilboum, R. (2006). Thiopurine S-methyltransferase pharmacogenetics: Insights, challenges and future directions. *Oncogene, 25*(11), 1629–1638. doi: 10.1038/sj.onc.1209372

Wu, Y. L., Zhou, C., Hu, C. P., Feng, J., Lu, S., Huang, Y., . . . Geater, S. L. (2014). Afatinib versus cisplatin plus gemcitabine for first-line treatment of Asian patients with advanced non-small-cell lung cancer harbouring EGFR mutations (LUX-Lung 6): An open-label, randomised phase 3 trial. *The Lancet Oncology, 15*(2), 213–222. doi: 10.1016/S1470-2045(13)70604-1

Xu, C. F., Reck, B. H., Xue, Z., Huang, L., Baker, K. L., Chen, M., & Pandite, L. (2010). Pazopanib-induced hyperbilirubinemia is associated with Gilbert's syndrome UGT1A1 polymorphism. *British Journal of Cancer, 102*(9), 1371–1377. doi: 10.1038/sj.bjc.6605653

Yan, M., Parker, B. A., Schwab, R., & Kurzrock, R. (2014). HER2 aberrations in cancer: Implications for therapy. *Cancer Treatment Reviews, 40*(6), 770–780. doi: 10.1016/j.ctrv.2014.02.008

Yokota, T. (2014). Is biomarker research advancing in the era of personalized medicine for head and neck cancer? *International Journal of Clinical Oncology, 19*(2), 211–219. doi: 10.1007/s10147-013-0660-4

Zanger, U. M., & Klein, K. (2013). Pharmacogenetics of cytochrome P450 2B6 (CYP2B6): Advances on polymorphisms, mechanisms, and clinical relevance. *Frontiers in Genetics, 4*, 24. doi: 10.3389/fgene.2013.00024

Zdanowicz, M. M., & American Society of Health-System Pharmacists. (2010). *Concepts in pharmacogenomics*. Bethesda, MD: American Society of Health-System Pharmacists.

Zhi, X., Zhou, X., Wang, W., & Xu, Z. (2013). Practical role of mutation analysis for imatinib treatment in patients with advanced gastrointestinal stromal tumors: A meta-analysis. *PLoS One, 8*(11), e79275. doi: 10.1371/journal.pone.0079275

Ethics and Patient Care

John Twomey, PhD, PNP, FNP

9

Ethical analysis of acts done in the biomedical sphere appears to be relatively straightforward. Established moral norms are based on accepted sociocultural beliefs and promulgated widely through professional education and popular media as well as traditional fonts of moral education, including family, religious, and educational institutions. Healthcare professionals are socialized into acceptance of familiar ethical values that are translated into rules for behavior and set forth in broad expectations, such as those contained in professional codes of ethics. Meanwhile, licensure and employment requirements insist on adherence to ethics-based rules.

A genetic counselor who has been raised within a protective and loyal family, has been educated within a system of schools that emphasizes human rights and dignity, and embraces the professional duty to protect the genetic information of clients, should have little problem not sharing the diagnosis of a genetic illness with family members for whom the client does not wish to disclose (Clarke et al., 2005). However, the complexities of this seemingly simple ethical question of nondisclosure causes moral self-examination in many circumstances (Dupras, Ravitsky, & Williams-Jones, 2012). Despite rules denoting that clients control their information within families, parties to disclosure decisions often can be put in positions where they discern that other parties within a family have such significant interest in the results of a genetic diagnosis that the profession does not simply honor the request for nondisclosure, instead putting significant efforts into

OBJECTIVES

- How does bioethical analysis of pharmacogenetic technologies needs to go beyond simplistic application of ethical principles to practice.

- Why are the ethical issues in the Nuffield Report on Ethics and Pharmacogenetics applicable in identifying ongoing pharmacogenomic issues?

- What are the current policies in the US that protect genomic information and what implications do these policies have for current and future pharmacogenetic practice.

- Articulate ethical issues that might arise as pharmacogenetic technologies are translated into clinical practice.

changing the client's mind about disclosure. This ongoing discussion about how to handle the complexities of sharing information has caused a paradigm shift in the genetic counseling field about the use of nondirective counseling that is both practice- and ethics-based (Elwyn, Gray, & Clarke, 2000; Weil et al., 2006).

Ethical analysis of any rule-based act goes beyond simply observing whether an individual acting within a professional relationship "follows the rule." Remember that the rules were put in place for a reason, usually to safeguard a right or interest that reasonable people believe needs to be protected. Most rules governing the practice of healthcare professionals are a mixture of both ethical and legal concerns, and many are context-driven. For example, a military member who is ordered to submit to a genetic diagnostic test may have fewer privacy rights regarding control of the results than his civilian counterpart (Baruch & Hudson, 2008).

The Method of Bioethical Analysis

How do we do ethical analysis of a biomedical action if we cannot simply assume its adherence to being "correct"? In actuality, such analysis is done all the time, and its methods are familiar to anyone working with the basic scientific method of inquiry.

Theory Generation

Although bioethical behaviors have been prescribed for many years, bioethical theory as we know it is relatively new. Our principle-based system of basing rules upon the cardinal precepts of autonomy, beneficence, nonmaleficence, and justice was presented in a unified system only within the past two generations of our current Western healthcare system. In response to several trends that included a greater recognition of human rights within society as well as an insistence that individuals be given greater control over their healthcare decisions, theorists from disciplines within religion, theology, and healthcare began to ponder how historical concepts about human dignity should be emphasized within the healthcare system. As revelations about past medical abuses in human subjects research as well as increases in medical technologies began to be discussed in the 1960s and 1970s, it was realized that decisions about issues such as extending life through machinery not only needed much input from the individuals involved in these decisions, but also needed some theoretical rationales for the behavior of actors in the healthcare system (Beauchamp & Childress, 2008).

Within the past half century, there has been a proliferation of attention to raising the profile of bioethical thought and action within the healthcare stage. Healthcare professionals have updated their codes (Fowler, 1999) or generated new ones as the adjunct healthcare professions have emerged. This trend has extended even to subspecialties within specific professions as people practicing with more knowledge of the specific mind or organ system determine that they have discrete obligations that others do not (Perlis & Shannon, 2012).

For example, the International Association of Nurses in Genetics (ISONG; www.isong. org/ISONG_position_statements.php) periodically publishes and updates position statements on clinical duties and ethical responsibilities. In papers addressing such topics as access to genomic healthcare, the need to safeguard genomic information, and issues related to consumer marketing of genetic tests, this specialty group has assumed the responsibility to facilitate better genomic nursing care.

Meanwhile, organizations also provide guidance and rules to follow for workers. For example, an organization that focuses on a specific service, such as end-of-life care, will define to its employees that an expected value is compassion and that interventions such as pain control meet more important clinical goals than other therapeutic actions (Boulanger, Ibarra, & Wagner, 2014). Organizations frequently will characterize these values as ethical imperatives that go beyond baseline professional bioethics. The patients/clients whose interests now go beyond simply needing to be passively protected are expected (as well as expecting) to participate in decision-making around their own care.

Given the fact that so many factors now affect the calculus of what is "correct" ethical behavior, it is quite reasonable that analyzing the ethics of a given healthcare phenomenon demands that observation of such a behavior and interpreting, rather than simple judging, is desirable and will help to move forward the practice of bioethical behavior. Therefore, the next step in the process would be to use the concepts of ethical theory, which continue to center around patient advocacy and justice, to help develop the questions to guide any observation and subsequent analysis.

Defining Questions to Ask and Analyze

It is not difficult to comprehend why we want to examine the behaviors of healthcare professionals and the outcomes of their actions through an ethical prism. Despite the belief that the vast majority of healthcare professionals act in ways that they intend to be entirely moral in nature, there are reasons why we cannot assume that the end result will be automatically pristine from an ethical perspective. The first reason is fairly obvious: There is an enormous amount of diversity of thought about what is right and wrong in the clinical setting. Disagreements can arise among professional groups (Gaudine, LeFort, Lamb, & Thorne, 2011), among patients making decisions (Quinn, Vadaparampil, King, Miree, & Friedman, 2009), or within groups (Butz, Redman, Fry, & Kolodner, 1998). Disagreements do not imply a right or wrong answer about the morality of a given action. By examining the actions of a given population, though, rationales can be given for decisions, such as when families' decisions do not consistently reflect the ethical guidelines of professional experts (Twomey, 2002).

A cardinal example of how examination of empirical data can provide insight into ethical behavior was seen by the reports of the SUPPORT Trial in the 1990s. The U.S. Patient Self Determination Act (PSDA) of 1990 provides patients with the tools to make end-of-life decisions, primarily through the encouragement of advance directives being executed after admission to hospitals (Teno et al., 1997). Results showed that despite the efforts of many healthcare personnel, people were still dying in pain while being subjected to extraordinary measures that they had not agreed to (The SUPPORT Investigators, 1995).

This example reflects aggregate numbers of actions that can be easily characterized as morally desirable or acceptable. What this example does not do, by any means, is explain why such behaviors exist. That takes another level of action, such as interventional programs based on studies such as the SUPPORT Trial.

A second reason for doing observation and analysis of clinical actions that have ethical import is the dynamic nature of healthcare, particularly the technological side of this very broad field. Specifically, in genetics, new capabilities in areas such as sequencing have provided lots of new data that have possible implications for clinical care, such as the discovery of new single nucleotide polymorphisms that seem to be linked with a given health issue, such as attention deficit disorder in children and adults. An ethical analysis that may be worthwhile could include the impact of discussing in public the possible link between gene and behavior and determining how the possibility of such a genetic linkage impacts behavior and clinical decision-making or policy changes. For example, many would support research into the genetic basis of attention deficit hyperactivity disorder (ADHD), but the possible implications of being labeled with the "ADHD gene" may give pause to those who might enroll their child in such research (Rothenberger, 2012).

Another rationale for ethical analysis is that when technologies emerge at a rapid pace, there is a concomitant rush to construct new inquiries into their use. Therefore, in genetic research, it has become a practice to collect genetic donations from research subjects in a trial about one topic, such as behavioral characteristics, but to preserve the specimens, often in repositories not under control of the original researcher, so that future, undefined research can be done using the original specimen (Beskow, 2014). Ethical analysis of the possible issues of such practices is deserved.

Genomic and Genetic Ethics

Ethical behavior in genomic and genetic healthcare has been viewed as a necessary area of observation and evaluation since the origins of the project to map the human genome. The Human Genome Project has consistently had funds specified within it to support the examination of emergent behaviors that new technologies facilitated regarding the human genome, both in the use of new knowledge and how new possibilities are being interpreted (Walker & Morrissey, 2013). This program and other funded and unfunded initiatives have kept the focus on almost all clinical initiatives involving genetic technologies within the past 15 years.

One example of a research study that examined consumer choices and allowed for ethical analysis involved the growing practice of direct-to-consumer advertising for genetic testing. When comparing the usage of genetic testing services for the BRCA mutation by consumers who were exposed (or not) to media-driven advertising offering the test (by the private company holding the patent for the specific testing technology), researchers found significantly higher rates of requests for testing in the markets where advertising was used, no matter what was the relative risk of the individuals in the aggregate groups (Mouchawar et al., 2005).

This example provides us with a worthwhile exercise in ethical analysis. Consider first the question of ethical responsibility. We have defined that unnecessary genetics services were accessed because certain patients —who were not at the level of risk that experts in hereditary breast cancer consider high enough to be tested—were encouraged to be tested. Obviously, the company offering the test put its interests ahead of those of the potential customers. Also, possibly scarce resources were misused given that genetics counselors in the markets where advertising occurred were overconsulted; thus, possible violations of justice and the duty of veracity occurred.

However, society has not determined that private companies, even those selling health-related products, have such ethical duties to their patients. Some may argue that by advertising the testing opportunity, potential patients who were at higher risk learned about testing opportunities that they did not know existed and sought necessary genetic counseling. Therefore, there may be counterbalancing enhancements of the exercise of autonomy and beneficence through allowing this practice, which actually is an example of a policy issue that has ethical implications.

Current Uses of Ethical Analysis in Genomic/Genetic Health Practices

Arguably, all decisions made in the healthcare sphere involve some ethical components due to their implications for effects on individual patient care. That seems to be the current state of the ethics of genomic healthcare. The promise of the Ethical, Legal, and Social Implications (ELSI) Program of the Human Genome Project appeared to be that because of the expectation that the unlocked secrets of the human genome would have revolutionary effects on healthcare, it was best to begin anticipating such effects by addressing them in order to maximize benefits and minimize harms (http://www.genome.gov/elsi/).

This fear of ethical ignorance about unanticipated genetic discoveries has not been realized, but not because of the prescient visions of the ELSI program: The greatest technological advances that emerged from the mapping of the genome did not involve new interventional capabilities, but centered on the improved methods of such mapping. Techniques such as computer-assisted microarray (Wang, Istepanian, & Yong Hua, 2003) allow for faster and more accurate studies of gene expression. However, the greatest strides have not been shared in the areas of patient therapies. Most uses of genomic technology involve greater and easier diagnostics for genetic contributions to disease, and less to therapeutics. Essentially, genomic research is still bridging between being exploratory and applied at this time.

Ethical Analysis in Pharmacogenomics: A Framework

Here are the two current areas of ethical analysis in pharmacogenomics:

- An analysis of issues that were projected during the early years of the Human Genome Project

- An analysis of possible derivative issues that could evolve as the field of pharmacogenomics becomes more clinically relevant

The other chapters in this book describe the current state of the science and practice in pharmacogenomics. Suffice it to say that as of this writing, the ethical issues that are current and could be analyzed have remained relatively stable over the past decade. A review of these issues is in order.

The Nuffield Report on Ethics and Pharmacogenetics

In 2003, the Nuffield Council on Bioethics issued a report entitled *Pharmacogenetics: Ethical Issues*. The council is a privately funded British think tank that examines scientific and ethical issues within the perspective of a group whose centralized healthcare system is run by a republican government and that provides universal care to its citizens. Based in the culture of Western and developed medicine, many of the council's values reflect those ideals and concerns of other developed countries, including the United States.

The basic technologic premises of the reports were that pharmacogenetic tests examined genes, chromosomes, or proteins and their responses to "a medicine" (Lipton, 2003). For the purposes of our discussion, the definition of "medicine" is expanded to include entities such as biologics or pharmaceuticals derived from immune system-based drugs. The group also noted that pharmacogenetics involved variation within people in how they processed medications, such as within the cytochrome P450 enzyme system for metabolizing many medications. Pharmacogenetics can also be a system of disease characterization, such as when an individual tumor's genome is examined to determine the most effective chemotherapy to employ. Also, pharmacogenetics was seen as a possible means of determining whether genetic diseases had variable responses to drugs so that doses could be altered, and the "one size fits all" practice that most practitioners employ in drug therapy could be improved to enlarge safety profiles and perhaps save money.

The report took an interesting angle on its analysis, which by its nature was futuristic. It used the perspective of *beneficence* as its primary prism to judge the ethical good of a pharmacogenetic intervention. From an ethical perspective, beneficence often is an individualistic principle and most easily measurable by the goods provided to a patient. Conversely, a *protectionist* perspective might deem that screening tests are critiqued by looking at the proportion of lives saved by such a test versus those who undergo treatment or further diagnostics because of false positive results. However, pharmacoge-nomics ethical analysis seems to lend itself naturally to look at beneficence and autonomy because of the tendency for people to assume the individuality of the single genome. Of course, this ignores the fact that of the 22,000 plus genes in the human genome, almost all are shared in some form and that our individuality comes in the expression of such genes after transcription and protein formation (Pertea & Salzberg, 2010).

The report made recommendations in three areas:

- Clinical care
- Clinical research
- Public policy

Each area had legitimate promise for genetic technological development at the time of the report in 2003, and each has had some interesting activities in the decade since. A varying amount of ethical discussion has occurred for all of the topics, but the level of effect that these developments and discussions on individual care and healthcare policy have has been rather minimal to date.

Clinical Care

The Nuffield Council accurately anticipated the biggest challenges that pharmacogenetics will provide ethically would emanate from the fact that any clinical implementation of new technologies would be significant only if accepted at the level of the practitioner and patient. Specifically, could the following actions be taken?

- Will pharmacogenomic information be developed to the point that it is both re-liable enough to be clinically relevant while also being understandable enough for healthcare professionals to use such information accurately and to convey the relevant data to the patients in comprehensible manners?
- Will pharmacogenetic technologies be developed so that access to clinically rel-evant information is readily available to the practitioner and patient?
- How should autonomous choices made by patients that are not genomically "correct" be handled (such as, if patients whose mutations indicate that they should take more expensive medications request a cheaper, less efficacious drug)?

- What data should be shared with an individual who has provided genetic material for examination in a clinical or research setting if said data is not specifically contributory to an ongoing diagnosis or to help determine risk to a known genetic illness?

Clinical Research

The report devoted a large amount of discussion to the topic of research protections for subjects. This was a necessary acceptance that genetic research was (and is) still in an embryonic state and that large numbers of subjects would be enrolling in clinical trials. Therefore, several topics were put on the table for consideration for ethical analysis.

- What should the role of pharmacogenetics be in generalized clinical trials?
- How should privacy of genomic samples be handled?
- How should clinical researchers obtain and store genetic data?
- How should aggregate data be shared with secondary investigators, and what protections should exist for this data?
- If there is a belief that pharmacogenetic research could boost the beneficial aspects of current drugs, how should such research be encouraged?
- What is the role of clinical validity of genetic data, particularly in the discussion of whether subjects have a right to that data?

Public Policy

There has never been any doubt in the mind of observers that increased genetic technologies and genomic knowledge would force reconsiderations of many healthcare policies. Because of the essential ethic of genetics—specifically, that we are exploring hidden secrets of human structure and functioning not only in the format of a grand model but also in individualistic detail not imagined until only very recently—it has been appreciated that the true power of such knowledge is how it is accessed, interpreted, and stored. The Nuffield Report made several recommendations on topics related to the area of policy.

- How should genetic tests be regulated so that trust in their safety and validity can be ensured?

- What ethical concerns regarding the equitable provision of healthcare after genomic information is accepted as basic may emerge, and how should these concerns be addressed?
- How should research into genetic differences by groups, particularly racial and ethnic, be conducted in order to avoid discrimination and stereotyping about health responses?

Protecting Genetic Information in the Post-Nuffield Era

A large part of controlling the unintended effects of new genetic knowledge derived from the testing of individuals will probably be a result of how well rules and policies are developed to provide appropriate access to such information while still providing the individual with the ability to protect that person's genomic/genetic data. Several specific policy initiatives in the United States address overall protection of genetic data collected within the healthcare system.

HIPAA

The Health Insurance Portability and Accountability Act (HIPAA) is almost 20 years old. This omnibus act—legislated by the U.S. Congress and signed into federal law by President William J. Clinton—addressed several areas of healthcare, including the right of consumers to maintain health insurance when changing jobs. Additionally, it has become best known for its restrictions on healthcare agencies and providers for how they handle individual client's health data (Slive & Cramer, 2012). Anyone working in healthcare within the past generation has been cautioned not to make any "HIPAA violations." The term "HIPAA violation" has become the slogan for a violation of patient confidentiality, so much so that healthcare workers often do not stop to process the ethical grounding for this protection and simply chalk it up to a bureaucratic rule with which they must comply. Nonetheless, few would argue that HIPAA has not helped to raise awareness of the need to protect patient data.

The original HIPAA legislation, however, had crucial gaps in its protection for genetic privacy. For example, it does not forbid insurers from making decisions on some pricing of plans based on genetic information, nor does it forbid said insurers from releasing the results of genetic tests to other parties (Huber & Vorhaus, 2011). This lack of protections provides an example of how laws often fail to cover all contingencies from a moral standpoint because of the legislative process, which demands compromises on political grounds. HIPAA has been amended to encompass genetic privacies, but these changes have been in response to protections dictated by the promulgation of the Genetic Information Nondiscrimination Act of 2008 (GINA; The Network for Public Health Law, 2013).

GINA

The Genetic Information Nondiscrimination Act (GINA) of 2008 provides an example of a directed effort to anticipate and prevent moral harms from arising due to the choices of patients who have legitimate interests in knowing their genomic health information. Six years after its implementation, it enjoys wide support in the United Sates due to the perceptions of consumers that the act properly protects genetic information while encouraging healthcare professionals to be part of the genetic counseling process (Almeling & Gadarian, 2014).

GINA has two main protections: total restriction on the use of genetic health information to make employment decisions and its equally strict prohibition on making genetic information a requirement for attaining health insurance. This also includes the use of genomic knowledge legitimately collected by the health insurance company (for example, maternal health history) to forbid coverage for another worthy applicant (for example, a child with an inherited genetic condition born to the mother; Steck & Eggert, 2011).

The passage of GINA appears to have been a response to a legitimate ethical problem in American healthcare. There was credible information to bolster the claim that genetic discrimination in employment and insurance applications was significant (Feldman, 2012). Probably the biggest issue with this discrimination was that although some of it could be documented, much of it was also rumor. Clinicians were, and remain, surprisingly unclear about the illegitimate use of genetic data and the scope of any sanctions, legal or otherwise, during the period before the passage of GINA and also the years subsequent to its passage (Laedtke, O'Neill, Rubinstein, & Vogel, 2012). This knowledge deficit is upsetting, because without reassurance from healthcare professionals, patients may avoid seeking genomic health resources, such as risk assessment, in fear that the risks from discrimination may outweigh the benefits of possible medical interventions.

Patient Protection and Affordable Care Act (PPACA)

Two years after the passage of the GINA, the Patient Protection and Affordable Care Act (PPACA, commonly referred to as simply "ACA") was enacted by the U.S. Congress. Although elements of the ACA affect genomic health, they are mostly indirect and complementary to HIPAA and GINA in regard to the provision and protection of genomic health services (Sarata, DeBergh, & Staman, 2011). The ACA actually would be insufficient on its own regarding ensuring access to genomic health services because it does not apply to self-insurers, whereas the scope of GINA extends to patients and not the insurers—a key point.

From an ethical viewpoint, though, the ACA makes a dramatic shift in the American perspective on genomic health. HIPAA and GINA address the protection of patient information after genomic testing and diagnosing have occurred and worries about misuse of such data can arise. This is an individualistic perspective and is rooted in our desire to protect an individual's autonomy: a condition that allows decisions to be as free from nongermane influences as possible, such as worries about a diagnosis affecting employability. The ACA could be a much more powerful ethical force moving forward because of its overarching goal of providing universal health coverage for American citizens. Although the act itself does not define all specific services to be provided, it does provide for a pluralistic participation in the process to define what should be provided to all patients (Skinner, 2013).

This movement to an ethic of justice is significant in genomic health. No one has ever claimed that the provision of genomic services was equitable, even in the area of the widest provision of such services: namely, the universal newborn screening program. However, most ethical conversations have been in the area of protection. Now, the discussion widens. Varying constituencies will weigh in on what genomic tests, screenings, and possible therapies are desirable, and negotiations will occur with insurers about what is to be paid for. This will be an incremental process, and no one would argue that answers about worthy services will be entirely science-based—but once determined, a given service will be available.

Availability will not necessarily mean universal accessibility. The ACA leaves choices about levels of coverage up to the insurers, states, and consumers. Unless a specific service is deemed essential for all, such as newborn screening, it is possible that a test will be offered but the necessary accompanying genetic counseling is not, unless an option exists to purchase the service through higher premiums or if a state covers the service as part of its Medicaid program.

An example about how the ACA may affect availability of genomic services would be if pharmaceuticals of a given class, such as antibiotics, routinely were found to have very detailed genetic profiles such that their pharmacokinetics and pharmacodynamics actions could be predicted with very high correlations. Several decisions about drug availability may be made that have cascading ethical implications:

- Empirical prescribing of antibiotics may cease as health plans routinely begin requiring genetic testing of patients. This would include baseline testing for information on drug absorption and metabolism, as well as individual serologicals for infective organisms when acute illness occurs.
- Unless rapid laboratory testing is available, patients may routinely have to wait to begin antibiotic therapy in nonemergent situations.
- Antibiotic use may subsequently drop, and pharmaceutical companies may find that producing these products is not cost-effective, so the price of low-cost therapies increases as their usage rates drop.
- Some insurance plans may begin to include the cost of acute genetic testing for microbe-specific antimicrobials under defined deductible ceiling costs that must be covered before full payment of such testing will be reimbursed by the insurance company.

One can see how in this scenario, in which technological advances provide a marvelous opportunity to move toward a personalized, genetic-based health service, the unintended consequences negatively impact many of those patients seeking such care. Many patients would have beneficial interventions restricted and their choices limited, not broadened. The concept of justice would be deranged, as many individuals who currently have access and significant need would have less care than now. A full ethical analysis would have to examine whether the restrictions produced enough aggregate goods to accept the limits on autonomous choice that would occur under such a discrete policy.

The Evolving Ethical Atmosphere in Genomic Health

No big ethical surprises have emerged in pharmacogenetics since the Nuffield Report was published. However, it is useful to look back at those issues identified and discuss the state of the ethical discourse particularly about pharmacogenetics. Very little empirical data has been produced on the topic, but that is a byproduct of the lack of progress in the technologies of pharmacogenetics.

Current Ethical Issues in Pharmacogenetics

In the three main areas identified by the Nuffield Report—public policy, clinical research, and clinical care—ethical themes tend to overlap. As seen, overall concerns about genetic discrimination have been somewhat addressed by legislation; however, such discrimination protections target specific types of actions based on genetic knowledge that are mostly economic and related to privacy. It remains to be seen how society will react to having more genomic health data available. Therefore, privacy itself should continue to be a specific goal of genomic healthcare, including pharmacogenomics. Several commentators have noted that pharmacogenetics progress has not presented us with a host of new ethical issues, but that as expected advances occur, this branch of scientific technology will challenge us with many convergent moral concerns (Marx-Stolting, 2007; Robertson, Brody, Buchanan, Kahn, & McPherson, 2002; Schubert, 2004).

> In the futuristic film *Gattaca,* the Western society depicted has officially outlawed genetic discrimination. However, easy access to the genetic information of self and others has created a culture where social mobility and employment status are directly tied into one's genome, reminding us of the importance of keeping privacy at the forefront of genomic healthcare.

Genetic Information: How Much to Collect, and Where Does It Go?

Collecting genetic data involves deepening the already invasive process that patients subject themselves to during the healthcare encounter. Beginning with the personal health history and moving into the family history, the clinician tries to collect enough information to paint as complete a picture as possible of the patient's genomic background before entering into the diagnostic phase of the process. By its nature, the gathering of personal data means harvesting information that is extraneous to the main goal of any clinical appointment, be it research or therapeutic. Advances in electronic health records (EHRs) make this process's collection and storage phases even more efficient. Because the diagnostic phase of the clinical encounter is deductive, often more information is sought during the process. If pharmacogenetic technology becomes ubiquitous in its involvement in clinical medicine, what are the implications?

A significant part of any discussion of patient information is availability and access. Although paper health records still exist in most clinical settings, the emergence of EHRs portend new challenges for the protection of patient information. From one perspective, the fact that such information may be password-protected may lead one to believe that this means that a layer of protection has been added beyond the simple locking of a file room door after hours. However, the fact that most EHRs are reliant on the Internet—and use of electronic information storage and servers—means that a goodly amount of data is available to skilled and determined hackers. Additionally, the use of portable computers and media makes such data theft a frightening reality in today's world (Schultz, 2012).

Stolen genetic information is probably at no more risk for abuse than other medical data because thieves are more interested in the financial and personal information contained in the record. Key details such as Social Security numbers and birthdates are often recorded together in the EHR and in insurance records. Credit information may be archived in other parts of the patient files, too. Are there any real personal threats to privacy that have increased because of possible pharmacogenetic advances?

It is hard to say that harms will occur more than benefits from privacy concerns that are directly attributable to pharmacogenetics. Most of the talk about emergent testing for genetic involvement in pharmacodynamics and pharmacokinetics assumes that uses will occur predominantly in prescription medications, such as antibiotics and chemotherapeutic agents.

A common occurrence in today's health market, however, is the movement of prescription medications being reclassified as over-the-counter (OTC) compounds. These drugs still need to carry pertinent patient information on their packaging. What if such information contains significant genetic information as one of its proscriptions? What if purchasers of medications are divided into two common groups: responders and nonresponders? Will pharmacies—which now provide immunizations and some primary care health services, including drug prescribing—become a place to have common genetic testing done? It is not beyond the realm of belief to imagine testing for Cytochrome p450 becoming rather common as the technology improves its time for results from days to perhaps hours. This could open the door to pharmacists being able to recommend testing for OTC medications such as proton pump inhibitors and nonsteroidal pain relievers (Samer, Lorenzini, Rollason, Daali, & Desmeules, 2013).

Simply carrying to the register a box of pills that identifies you as a heterozygous allele carrier of a given gene to those with some genetic knowledge does not appear to put one at great risk. We all have had to carry personal care items around the drug store, and the level of embarrassment this exposed us to is a matter of personal feelings. Perhaps the privacy risk from increasing the genomic data entering one's health record is no greater than that of other forms of health data.

Who Deserves What Information?

Very few medical screening or diagnostic tests provide data that is specific to only one possible health condition. Because of the polymorphic nature of one's phenotype, the genetic structure being examined for one health issue may have implications for other health conditions. But the key issue of being surprised when requesting a genetic test when one is a competent adult can be defused by thorough preparation during the consent process. However, what if the subject of the test is incompetent by age?

Testing children for late-onset genetic illnesses has been the focus of debate for many years (Caga-anan, Smith, Sharp, & Lantos, 2012; Rhodes, 2006; Twomey, Bove, & Cassidy, 2008). Arguments that parents should not have knowledge about a child's health for which there is no intervention and in which symptoms may not even occur until adulthood have been countered by claims that parents are the best counselors to their children and that the parents need the diagnostic information to reassure themselves emotionally, especially when the particular illness appears within the family history. There is no consensus about how to move forward on a strict policy that supports the recommendations to delay such testing, and presumably, most genetic services support the final family decision.

Does pharmacogenetics extend this concern? Although we have no good examples at this time of readily available genetic tests for common non-single gene late-onset conditions, it is conceivable that some such testing of interests to parents may be developed. Already, some single nucleotide polymorphisms (SNPs) have been linked with Type 2 diabetes mellitus, which might be modifiable through lifestyle changes (Howson et al., 2011), and other studies have linked SNPs with multiple mental health behavioral disorders (Hemmings et al., 2004). It is imaginable that arguments used in requests for late-onset genetic testing in children by parents may be repeated, and this may be disturbing in connection with disorders that have known pharmaceutical responses.

For instance, pediatric behavioral diagnosis and treatment are controversial. Because the behaviors involved may lead the individuals involved in a child's care to make different assessments, the use of genetic testing may be attractive for diagnosis and treatment (Patel & Barzman, 2013). It is not too difficult to imagine scenarios where parents who have had one child successfully treated for a childhood psychiatric illness request testing for a sibling based on the fact that validated genetic testing helped confirm the first child's diagnosis and suggested his pharmaceutical treatment based on equally validated pharmacogenetic testing. How far does the concept "It runs in the family" go? Should an asymptomatic child of any age be forced to undergo testing for a disease that may not present for years and possibly begin medication under the belief that the disease could be prevented?

This becomes a particularly acute problem in the research setting where the ethic is not beneficence but protection. Under the current Code of Federal Regulations 45 CFR 46, Subpart D, would a child with an asymptomatic psychiatric genetic diagnosis come under the auspices of 46.405 or 46.406? The former paragraph is for children generally considered ill, and the latter addresses healthy children and is assumed to offer more protections. Given that few children refuse to assent to participation in any trials that their parents seek to enroll them in (Caga-anan, et al., 2012), there might be a basis to consider new protections for children involved in pharmacogenetic trials or even drug trials based on their genotype (Holder, 2008).

Pharmacogenetic Drug Research

The volume of information now available through the ongoing study of the human genome has spurred scientists to consider a genetic component of almost any clinical issue that collects biological samples. Whether such research seeks to investigate biological or behavioral responses and illnesses, there has been an acceptance in health sciences research that "the future is now." This means that because of the anticipated continued expansion of genetic research technologies, it is best to "sample now, study later." By storing the genetic samples of research subjects who are enrolled in studies that are both genetic and nongenetic in nature, scientists are preparing for questions that may not even be conceptualized yet. However, such practices raise many ethical issues related to pharmacogenetic research (Caulfield, 2008).

Banking newborn tissue after testing the samples for nonsymptomatic diseases under a newborn screening program highlights many of the concerns about how genetic research is carried out (Ries, 2010). A large cohort of minor children is sampled under the acknowledgement that only a few will benefit. The consent process from parents is not rigorous. Few parents understand that the samples will be saved for future research. The children probably will never know. What duties are owed to these children? What if future studies discover remedies that could help the children? Should they be given the information necessary to take advantage of this new therapeutic knowledge? What if the benefit is simply that they would not have to undergo future pharmacogenetic testing because of the previous provision of their genetic material?

Subject Rights and Biobanking

Determining how much clinical research in pharmacogenetics is being done at this time is difficult. One recent article optimistically described the field as "burgeoning," but the listings provided of active trials was limited and did not seem to have many trials that actively linked genetic testing with specific genes or allele groups. The authors also noted that at this time, the U.S. Food & Drug Administration (FDA) will review submitted pharmacogenomic information on drugs but does not require such data when it reviews new applications (Beitelshees & Veenstra, 2011). The state of the art is probably best described by Limaye (2013), who noted that drug companies are storing much information on candidate SNPs but are not conducting many pharmacogenetic trials.

Clinical research ethics, in response to the HIV/AIDS pandemic, underwent a paradigm shift in the 1980s and 1990s. Whereas traditionally, the subject in a trial was a passive figure who was owed nothing from the researcher beyond reasonable protections from foreseeable harms, HIV and AIDS sufferers sought more when solicited to enroll in clinical trials. They refused to be randomized into possible placebo arms of trials, they insisted on being part of the planning of protocols, and they also negotiated up-front access to successful drugs even after the trial ended (Shilts, 1987).

Since this foundational era of research ethics, a fundamental shift toward treating the subject more as a partner in the investigation, with the researcher owing more duties than simple protections, has become more accepted (Boulanger et al., 2014). This shift has significant implication for the clinical research ethics in pharmacogenetics. For the most part, in the past, clinical researchers were looking for information that was gleaned from the responses of the patient. After individual responses were put into an aggregate pool, the client's participation was done unless some residual tissue was left over for future research. Now we are in an era where, in a significant amount of trials—even those in which genetic research is not the primary focus—genetic material is being taken from subjects, but with their consent. Quite often, as explained to the subject, such material is simply held for future use in case genetic technologies provide opportunities for inquiry in which this genetic material may be usefully studied.

The nature of this material is much different from traditional tissue donation. Because the genetic information available from a research tissue sample is not just a snapshot, but through amplification can reveal the entire individual phenotype, it provides an almost unending, immortal source of data. Genetic research samples are commonly stored at either the lab affiliated with the research institution or at regional biobanks whose main purpose is to warehouse genetic and other tissue specimens for collaborative research (Kang et al., 2013). Estimates placed the number of biological samples in 2007 at 270 million with expectations of 20 million samples being added to United States biobanks annually (Haga & Beskow, 2008). Because of the cost of doing research, some biobanks are reporting underuse of the samples on hand (Kang et al., 2013).

The core ethical issue involved in research using genetic samples is what is due to the subjects, all of whom are asked for generalized consent for their samples to be kept but probably don't realize that the use of their material may be years later and in research not even conceptualized at the time of donation. This includes pharmacogenetic research. Commentators have debated whether subjects who provided such genetic material are owed anything from the results of studies using their samples. It could be a benefit if subjects receive detailed information about their genome, if that information could have clinical significance (Ravitsky & Wilfond, 2006). Countering responses note that current levels of data that could affect clinical care are very low and are more likely to be a source of confusion. Additionally, given that the current guidelines for harvesting and storing such genetic material require de-identifying discrete samples to guarantee anonymity, it would put the promise of confidentiality at risk to maintain the link necessary to return information to the donors (Dressler & Juengst, 2006).

Ethnic and Racial Discrimination Concerns

Healthcare providers are pragmatists: If they find a useful intervention, and it is economically available to their individual patients, they usually will embrace it. The use of race to develop pharmacogenetically accurate drugs such as BiDil (isosorbide dinitrate/hydralazine hydrochloride) for use in congestive heart failure in African Americans and presumably other Black people, would seem appropriate. However, race turns out to be a varying factor in pharmacogenetic responses; and when clinicians see the marketing practices of drug companies who target groups for use of a drug, they may worry about the use of pharmacogenetic drug research (Kahn, 2006).

Part of the concern about race and ethnicity in pharmacogenetic research is because of the possibility that social implications of identifying particular groups with specific illness can cause a narrative that has negative implications about a group or can force individuals to be placed into a disease group instead of being treated individually (Phelan, Link, & Feldman, 2013). Members of American society who are from diverse groups as racial minorities and healthcare professionals themselves reflect both hope and concern about the use of targeted genetic research for interventions and pharmacogenetics (Idemyor, 2012; Ngui, Warner, & Roberts, 2014; Powell-Young & Spruill, 2013). Efforts must be taken to raise awareness about the multifactorial aspect of most genetic illness, and developing pharmacogenetic interventions should be about inclusivity, not exclusion.

Barriers to Clinical Utility

Several key ethical issues that may serve to slow the implementation of pharmacogenetic care in the clinical setting involve the human element that must interact with the technology that evolves.

Clinician Competency and Willingness

Although most Western healthcare practitioners work within an amazingly complex high-tech environment, individual practitioners are not necessarily early adopters of new technologies. The integration of genomic pharmacogenetics into current practices involves a variety of new challenges for clinicians, including:

- Learning new means of diagnostic interviewing and testing
- Understanding the subtleties of genetic pharmacodynamics and pharmacokinetics
- Translating this data back to the patient in an accurate and meaningful fashion

Clinical competence is a vital component of ethical professional practice. At this time, it is difficult to assume that genetic and genomic healthcare has moved into mainstream care. It still is viewed as a specialized area of healthcare. Although some healthcare practitioners are becoming more comfortable with integrating genomic care in their practices (Hoop, Roberts, Hammond, & Cox, 2008), many general practitioners in medicine and nursing are perhaps being prepared adequately during their basic education to feel knowledgeable enough to be proficient in basic genomic health but not advanced interventions, like pharmacogenetic care (Guttmacher, Porteous, & McInerney, 2007).

Professional organizations must renew their efforts to urge educational and accreditation bodies to require genomic/genetic health to be core subject areas in basic healthcare education. In the meantime, continued education in these areas must be a focal point for regulators and healthcare employers.

How Far Does Personalized Medicine Go? Disclosure to Third Parties

As testing capabilities for diagnostic and risk of genetic illnesses have increased, and healthcare professionals have had to include family history as a core part of the diagnostic process, they have had to consider the question about the interests of family members who clearly share genotypic features. This worry is particularly acute when a patient is diagnosed with a genomic issue that an at-risk family member clearly would have a significant interest in investigating. This is magnified when suddenly myriad therapeutic options are potentially opened for a family unit. One thing we have not considered openly in this chapter is that instituting a pharmacogenetic regimen involves necessary genetic testing. The question of what genetic information should be shared with family members has been discussed widely without any resolution. Only two legal cases have suggested a very limited obligation to share such information (Schleiter, 2009).

Generally, the issue of disclosure of private health information is forbidden legally and ethically and, therefore, is not an issue. Also, one can argue that although it may be a moral responsibility for a sibling to share family genotype information within the family group, this obligation does not spill over to the healthcare clinician. This view is supported by our professional ethical codes. However, society is increasingly beginning to show a willingness to force other types of health information to be shared, such as when a threat to a third party is voiced to a healthcare professional or a concern about a general danger to society becomes evident during an otherwise privileged conversation. The U.S. Department of Health and Human Services (2013) has issued a ruling that it is not a HIPAA violation to report such a threat. To be clear, at this time, the disclosure of genomic health information—whether diagnostic or pharmacogenetic in nature—is strictly protected (www.hhs.gov/ocr/privacy/hipaa/faq/ferpa_and_hipaa/520.html). However, the practitioner should be aware of evolving policies in this area that may be developed.

Summary

Pharmacogenetics does not present new ethical issues but highlights many of our traditional concerns about confidentiality, patient autonomy, and justice. Clinicians have the obligation to begin treating genomic healthcare as part of primary care, rather than as a subspecialty. This approach will allow pharmacogenomic healthcare to enter the mainstream of our medical system, and then we can begin examining how society views pharmacogenetics and how its practice should be modified so that all within our society can benefit from its practice.

Questions

Discuss whether increases in pharmacogenomic technologies have provided us with new ethical challenges or just presented us with new examples of older ethical issues.

Which of the following U.S. legislative acts affects the protection of personal genetic information?

    a. HIPAA

    b. GINA

    c. ACA

    d. All the above *

Which of the following U.S. legislative acts is the strongest law for the protection of personal genetic information?

    a. HIPAA

    b. GINA*

    c. ACA

References

Almeling, R., & Gadarian, S. K. (2014). Public opinion on policy issues in genetics and genomics. *Genetics in Medicine, 16*(6), 491–494. doi: 10.1038/gim.2013.175

Baruch, S., & Hudson, K. (2008). Civilian and military genetics: Nondiscrimination policy in a post-GINA world. *The American Journal of Human Genetics, 83*(4), 435–444. doi: 10.1016/j.ajhg.2008.09.003

Beauchamp, T., & Childress, J. (2008). *Principles of biomedical ethics* (6th ed.). New York, NY: Oxford University Press.

Beitelshees, A. L., & Veenstra, D. L. (2011). Evolving research and stakeholder perspectives on pharmacogenomics. *Journal of the American Medical Association, 306*(11), 1252–1253. doi: 10.1001/jama.2011.1343

Beskow, L. M., Dombeck, C. B., Thompson, C. P., Watson-Ormond, J. K., & Weinfurt, K. P. (2014). Informed consent for biobanking: consensus-based guidelines for adequate comprehension. *Genet Med.* doi: 10.1038/gim.2014.102

Boulanger, R. F., Ibarra, K., & Wagner, F. (2014). A road map to building ethics capacity in the home and community care and support services sector. *Healthcare Quarterly, 17*(1), 48–53.

Butz, A. M., Redman, B. K., Fry, S. T., & Kolodner, K. K. (1998). Ethical conflicts experienced by certified pediatric nurse practitioners in ambulatory settings. *Journal of Pediatric Health Care, 12*(4), 183–190.

Caga-anan, E. C. F., Smith, L., Sharp, R. R., & Lantos, J. D. (2012). Testing children for adult-onset genetic diseases. *Pediatrics, 129*(1), 163–167. doi: 10.1542/peds.2010-3743

Caulfield, T., McGuire, A. L., Cho, M., Buchanan, J. A., Burgess, M. M., Danilczyk, U., . . . Timmons, M. (2008). Research ethics recommendations for whole-genome research: consensus statement. *PLoS Biol, 6*(3), e73. doi: 10.1371/journal.pbio.0060073

Clarke, A., Richards, M., Kerzin-Storrar, L., Halliday, J., Young, M. A., Simpson, S. A., Stewart, H. (2005). Genetic professionals' reports of nondisclosure of genetic risk information within families. *European Journal of Human Genetics, 13*(5), 556–562. doi: 10.1038/sj.ejhg.5201394

Dressler, L. G., & Juengst, E. T. (2006). Thresholds and boundaries in the disclosure of individual genetic research results. *American Journal of Bioethics, 6*(6), 18–20; author reply W10–12. doi: 10.1080/15265160600934830

Dupras, C., Ravitsky, V., & Williams-Jones, B. (2012). Epigenetics and the environment in bioethics. *Bioethics 28*(7), 327–334. doi: 10.1111/j.1467-8519.2012.02007.x

Elwyn, G., Gray, J., & Clarke, A. (2000). Shared decision making and non-directiveness in genetic counselling. *Journal of Medical Genetics, 37*(2), 135–138. doi: 10.1136/jmg.37.2.135

Feldman, E. A. (2012). The Genetic Information Nondiscrimination Act (GINA): Public policy and medical practice in the age of personalized medicine. *Journal of General Internal Medicine, 27*(6), 743–746. doi: 10.1007/s11606-012-1988-6

Fowler, M. D. (1999). Relic or resource? The code for nurses. *American Journal of Nursing, 99*(3), 56–57.

Gaudine, A., LeFort, S. M., Lamb, M., & Thorne, L. (2011). Clinical ethical conflicts of nurses and physicians. *Nursing Ethics, 18*(1), 9–19. doi: 10.1177/0969733010385532

Guttmacher, A. E., Porteous, M. E., & McInerney, J. D. (2007). Educating health-care professionals about genetics and genomics. *Nature Reviews Genetics, 8*(2), 151–157.

Haga, S. B., & Beskow, L. M. (2008). Ethical, legal, and social implications of biobanks for genetics research. *Advances in Genetics, 60*, 505–544. doi: 10.1016/s0065-2660(07)00418-x

Hemmings, S. M. J., Kinnear, C. J., Lochner, C., Niehaus, D. J. H., Knowles, J. A., Moolman-Smook, J. C.,

. . . Stein, D. J. (2004). Early- versus late-onset obsessive–compulsive disorder: Investigating genetic and clinical correlates. *Psychiatry Research, 128*(2), 175–182. doi: http://dx.doi.org/10.1016/j.psychres.2004.05.007

Holder, A. R. (2008). Research with adolescents: Parental involvement required? *Journal of Adolescent Health, 42*(1), 1–2.

Hoop, J. G., Roberts, L. W., Hammond, K. A. G., & Cox, N. J. (2008). Psychiatrists' attitudes, knowledge, and experience regarding genetics: A preliminary study. *Genetics in Medicine, 10*(6), 439–449.

Howson, J. M. M., Rosinger, S., Smyth, D. J., Boehm, B. O., ADBW-END Study Group, & Todd, J. A. (2011). Genetic analysis of adult-onset autoimmune diabetes. *Diabetes, 60*(10), 2645–2653. doi: 10.2337/db11-0364

Huber, S., & Vorhaus, D. (2011). Genetic bill of rights proposed in Massachusetts. *Genomics Law Report.* Retrieved from http://www.genomicslawreport.com/index.php/2011/02/14/genetic-bill-of-rights-proposed-in-massachusetts/#more-5261

Idemyor, V. (2012). Genomic medicine: Health care issues and the unresolved ethical and social dilemmas. *American Journal of Therapeutics.* Advance online publication. doi: 10.1097/MJT.0b013e3182583bd1

Kahn, J. (2006). Race, pharmacogenomics, and marketing: Putting BiDil in context. *American Journal of Bioethics, 6*(5), W1–5. doi: 10.1080/15265160600755789

Kang, B., Park, J., Cho, S., Lee, M., Kim, N., Min, H., . . . Han, B. (2013). Current status, challenges, policies, and bioethics of biobanks. *Genomics & Informatics, 11*(4), 211–217. doi: 10.5808/gi.2013.11.4.211

Laedtke, A. L., O'Neill, S. M., Rubinstein, W. S., & Vogel, K. J. (2012). Family physicians' awareness and knowledge of the Genetic Information Non-Discrimination Act (GINA). *Journal of Genetic Counseling, 21*(2), 345–352. doi: 10.1007/s10897-011-9405-6

Limaye, N. (2013). Pharmacogenomics, theranostics and personalized medicine—the complexities of clinical trials: Challenges in the developing world. *Applied & Translational Genomics, 2,* 17–21. doi: http://dx.doi.org/10.1016/j.atg.2013.05.002

Lipton, P. (2003). Nuffield Council on bioethics consultation. *Pharmacogenomics, 4*(1), 91–95. doi: 10.1517/phgs.4.1.91.22585

Marx-Stolting, L. (2007). Pharmacogenetics and ethical considerations: Why care? *The Pharmacogenomics Journal, 7*(5), 293–296. doi: 10.1038/sj.tpj.6500425

Mouchawar, J., Hensley-Alford, S., Laurion, S., Ellis, J., Kulchak-Rahm, A., Finucane, M. L., . . . Ritzwoller, D. (2005). Impact of direct-to-consumer advertising for hereditary breast cancer testing on genetic services at a managed care organization: A naturally-occurring experiment. *Genetics in Medicine, 7*(3), 191–197. doi: 10.109701.gim.0000156526.16967.7a

The Network for Public Health Law. (2013). Regulatory changes to HIPAA under HITECH and GINA. Retrieved from https://www.networkforphl.org/_asset/y44fj6/HIPAA_fact-sheet2-20-13.pdf

Ngui, E. M., Warner, T. D., & Roberts, L. W. (2014). Perceptions of African-American health professionals and community members on the participation of children and pregnant women in genetic research. *Public Health Genomics, 17*(1), 23–32. doi: 10.1159/000355359

Patel, B. D., & Barzman, D. H. (2013). Pharmacology and pharmacogenetics of pediatric ADHD with associated aggression: A review. *Psychiatric Quarterly, 84*(4), 407–415. doi: 10.1007/s11126-013-9253-7

Perlis, C., & Shannon, N. (2012). Role of professional organizations in setting and enforcing ethical norms. *Clinics in Dermatology, 30*(2), 156–159. doi: 10.1016/j.clindermatol.2011.06.002

Pertea, M., & Salzberg, S. L. (2010). Between a chicken and a grape: Estimating the number of human genes. *Genome Biology, 11*(5), 206. doi: 10.1186/gb-2010-11-5-206

Phelan, J. C., Link, B. G., & Feldman, N. M. (2013). The genomic revolution and beliefs about essential racial differences: A backdoor to eugenics? *American Sociological Review, 78*(2), 167–191. doi: 10.1177/0003122413476034

Powell-Young, Y. M., & Spruill, I. J. (2013). Views of Black nurses toward genetic research and testing. *Journal of Nursing Scholarship, 45*(2), 151–159. doi: 10.1111/jnu.12015

Quinn, G. P., Vadaparampil, S. T., King, L. M., Miree, C. A., & Friedman, S. (2009). Conflict between values and technology: Perceptions of preimplantation genetic diagnosis among women at increased risk for hereditary breast and ovarian cancer. *Familial Cancer, 8*(4), 441–449.

Ravitsky, V., & Wilfond, B. S. (2006). Disclosing individual genetic results to research participants. *American Journal of Bioethics, 6*(6), 8–17. doi: 10.1080/15265160600934772

Rhodes, R. (2006). Why test children for adult-onset genetic diseases? *Mount Sinai Journal of Medicine, 73*(3), 609–616.

Ries, N. M., LeGrandeur, J., & Caulfield, T. (2010). Handling ethical, legal and social issues in birth cohort studies involving genetic research: responses from studies in six countries. *BMC Med Ethics, 11,* 4. doi: 10.1186/1472-6939-11-4

Robertson, J. A., Brody, B., Buchanan, A., Kahn, J., & McPherson, E. (2002). Pharmacogenetic challenges for the health care system. *Health Affairs, 21*(4), 155–167.

Rothenberger, L. G. (2012). Molecular genetics research in ADHD: ethical considerations concerning patients' benefit and resource allocation. *Am J Med Genet B Neuropsychiatr Genet, 159b*(8), 885–895. doi: 10.1002/ajmg.b.32111

Samer, C. F., Lorenzini, K. I., Rollason, V., Daali, Y., & Desmeules, J. A. (2013). Applications of CYP450 testing in the clinical setting. *Molecular Diagnosis & Therapy, 17*(3), 165–184. doi: 10.1007/s40291-013-0028-5

Sarata, M., DeBergh, J., & Staman, J. (2011). Congressional Research Service, The Genetic Information Nondiscrmination Act of 2008 and the Patient Protection Affordable Care Act of 2010: Overview and legal analysis of potential interactions. Washington, DC: Congressional Research Service.

Schleiter, K. E. (2009). A physician's duty to warn third parties of hereditary risk. *Virtual Mentor, 11*(9), 697–700. doi: 10.1001/virtualmentor.2009.11.9.hlaw1-0909

Schubert, L. (2004). Ethical implications of pharmacogenetics—do slippery slope arguments matter? *Bioethics, 18*(4), 361–378.

Schultz, D. (2012). As patients records go digital, theft and hacking problems grow. Retrieved from http://www.kaiserhealthnews.org/Stories/2012/June/04/electronic-health-records-theft-hacking.aspx

Shilts, R. (1987). *And the band played on*. New York, NY: St. Martin's Press.

Skinner, D. (2013). Defining medical necessity under the Patient Protection and Affordable Care Act. *Public Administration Review, 73,* S49–S59. doi: 10.2307/42003021

Slive, L., & Cramer, R. (2012). Health reform and the preservation of confidential health care for young adults. *The Journal of Law, Medicine & Ethics, 40*(2), 383–390. doi: 10.1111/j.1748-720X.2012.00671.x

Steck, M. B., & Eggert, J. A. (2011). The need to be aware and beware of the genetic information nondiscrimination act. *Clinical Journal of Oncology Nursing, 15*(3), E34–41. doi: 10.1188/11.cjon.e34-e41

The SUPPORT Investigators. (1995). A controlled trial to improve care for seriously ill hospitalized patients. The study to understand prognoses and preferences for outcomes and risks of treatments (SUPPORT). *Journal of the American Medical Association, 274*(20), 1591–1598.

Teno, J., Lynn, J., Wenger, N., Phillips, R. S., Murphy, D. P., Connors, A. F., Jr., . . . Knaus, W. A. (1997).

Advance directives for seriously ill hospitalized patients: Effectiveness with the patient self-determination act and the SUPPORT intervention. SUPPORT Investigators study to understand prognoses and preferences for outcomes and risks of treatment. *Journal of the American Geriatrics Society, 45*(4), 500–507.

Twomey, J. G. (2002). Genetic testing of children: Confluence or collision between parents and professionals? *AACN Clinical Issues, 13*(4), 557–566.

Twomey, J. G., Bove, C., & Cassidy, D. (2008). Presymptomatic genetic testing in children for neurofibromatosis 2. *Journal of Pediatric Nursing, 23*(3), 183–194.

Walker, R. L., & Morrissey, C. (2013). Bioethics methods in the ethical, legal, and social implications of the human genome project literature. *Bioethics*. Advance online publication. doi: 10.1111/bioe.12023

Wang, X. H., Istepanian, R. S. H., & Yong Hua, S. (2003). Microarray image enhancement by denoising using stationary wavelet transform. *IEEE Transactions on NanoBioscience, 2*(4), 184–189. doi: 10.1109/TNB.2003.816225

Weil, J., Ormond, K., Peters, J., Peters, K., Biesecker, B. B., & LeRoy, B. (2006). The relationship of nondirectiveness to genetic counseling: Report of a workshop at the 2003 NSGC Annual Education Conference. *Journal of Genetic Counseling, 15*(2), 85–93. doi: 10.1007/s10897-005-9008-1

Pharmacogenomics/ Pharmacogenetics and Interprofessional Education and Practice

10

Gayle Brazeau, PhD

Pharmacogenetics and pharmacogenomics are areas where interprofessional education and practice can easily be developed and implemented throughout our professional curriculums and across practice sites. Integration of knowledge, critical-thinking skills, and communication skills associated with pharmacogenetics and pharmacogenomics concepts will be essential to all future healthcare practitioners, particularly with the development of personalized disease and medicine identified through enhanced genetic screening in patients.

Nursing students and nurses can and must play a critical role in working with their patients and families to understand how these elements have an effect on care and treatment. The profession of nursing, both entry-level practitioners and advanced practitioners, can play an essential role with other healthcare professionals to optimize patient wellness and care through involvement in interprofessional educational opportunities in our health science programs and through patient-centered teams in practice sites.

OBJECTIVES

- Interprofessional competencies in healthcare can be integrated into classrooms and clinics when delivering team-based patient-centered care.
- The linkages of pharmacogenetics and pharmacogenomics with interprofessional competencies are essential.
- Pharmacogenetics and pharmacogenomics are an excellent foundation to collaborate with other healthcare professionals through the interprofessional competency domains.
- Nursing education at all levels must include contemporary pharmacogenetics and pharmacogenomics concepts and technologies.

Nursing has certainly been a key player in advancing interprofessional education through its efforts in promoting and enhancing the opportunities for the use of simulations in health science programs (American Association of Colleges of Nursing, 2006, 2008, 2011; Cronenwett et al., 2007, 2009). Nursing education since 2006 has embraced the expectations for interprofessional collaboration behaviors as essentials for baccalaureate, master's, and doctoral education, as well as using the Institute of Medicine framework for the core competencies in their efforts for pre-licensure and graduate competency statements emphasizing quality and safety outcomes as well as team-based competencies and teamwork (American Association of Colleges of Nursing, 2006, 2008, 2011; National Research Council, 2003).

The May 2011 report from the Interprofessional Education Collaborative (IPEC), which included representatives from the American Association of Colleges of Nursing, the American Association of Colleges of Osteopathic Medicine, the American Association of Colleges of Pharmacy, the American Dental Education Association, the Association of American Medical Colleges, and the Association of Schools of Public Health, provides the vision and insights into how pharmacogenetics and pharmacogenomics have and will continue to be essential to interprofessional team-based care (IPEC, 2011).

Interprofessional competencies in healthcare can easily be implemented and integrated in our classrooms and clinics when considering the important role of pharmacogenetics and pharmacogenomics in delivering team-based patient centered care.

Interprofessional Principles and Pharmacogenetics/ Pharmacogenomics

The core competencies for interprofessional collaborative practice provide an excellent framework for developing educational programs and practice that center around pharmacogenetics and pharmacogenomics (Interprofessional Education Collaborative Expert Panel, 2011). The principles of interprofessional competencies and their essential linkages to pharmacogenetics and pharmacogenomics are:

- **Patient-centered care:** Each patient is unique in his/her genetic background.
- **Community/population-oriented care:** Understanding differences in pharmacogenetics of communities or populations can provide insight into cultural

differences. Healthcare professionals must realize the importance of epigenetics in health, wellness, and patient care.

- **Relationship-focused care:** Healthcare professionals, particularly those involved with direct patient care, must focus on maintaining the best patient care and positive patient interactions even if they know specific pharmacogenetics of the patient.

- **Process-oriented:** Healthcare professionals must have the knowledge foundations and critical-thinking skills to understand new technologies centered on pharmacogenetics and pharmacogenomics and their input on patient care.

- **Linked to learning activities, educational strategies, and behavioral assessments that are developmentally appropriate for the learner:** Educational programs for new healthcare professionals and continuing education programs must be competency-based and involve demonstration of competencies.

- **Integrated learning across the professional career:** Healthcare practitioners must continue to enhance their clinical knowledge and skills as related to pharmacogenetics and pharmacogenomics because this will become more important in optimizing patient-centered care. Continuing professional development programs must include pharmacogenetics and pharmacogenomics concepts.

- **Sensitive to the systems context/applicable across practice settings:** Pharmacogenetics and pharmacogenomics will be involved with each patient across all the life stages and in all practice settings, as well as community and population health.

- **Applicable across all healthcare professions:** With patient-centered care at the core, all healthcare professionals must realize the effect of pharmacogenetics, pharmacogenomics, and epigenetics in their own interactions with the patient and in their team interactions.

- **Stated in language common and meaningful across the professions:** The language of genetics and genomics is essential to patient-centered team-based care. Individuals on the healthcare team must understand genetic terms and technologies.

- **Outcome-driven decision-making:** Using pharmacogenetics and pharmacogenomics for each patient can form the foundation for rational decision-making to optimize patient health and wellness and optimize desired clinical outcomes.

Genetics and Treatment Decisions

An individual's genetics influences wellness and health issues throughout that individual's life cycle. Technologies for improved testing throughout the life cycle, in the clinic or at the bedside, will continue to advance identifying an individual's genetic makeup and examining its interaction with the environment.

The challenge for the healthcare professional is that the link between an individual's genetic makeup and disease is often unclear: We only know a few diseases that are associated with a single gene. It therefore becomes critical for nurses and other healthcare professionals to understand and speak the same language: for example, whether a disease is autosomal recessive or autosomal dominant, x-linked recessive or x-linked dominant, or y-linked. Also, nurses and other healthcare professionals need to know the effect of these polymorphisms on families regarding inheritance, as to whether the disease will affect males and females equally or is sex-linked.

Examples of autosomal recessive genes leading to disease include phenylketonuria (PKU) and cystic fibrosis. Autosomal dominant genes leading to disease include Huntington's disease and myotonic dystrophy Type 1 and can potentially affect males and females in families equally. Duchenne muscular dystrophy is an example of an x-linked recessive disease resulting in progressive proximal muscular dystrophy affecting males. Rett syndrome is an x-linked dominant neurodevelopment disorder occurring predominantly in females (Chial, 2008). An individual's genetic makeup, certainly, is not the only factor that a healthcare professional needs to consider when working to enhance health and wellness of individuals or their community. Environmental factors have and continue to influence wellness and health issues. Epigenetics, or the modification of gene expression independent of the gene sequence, does play a key role in health, wellness, and disease. Environmental factors or influences can affect an individual's heritable traits. As such, our culture and living environments must always be considered by healthcare teams when promoting health and wellness as well as in the treatment of disease. Genetics and epigenetics should be important components focusing on the relationship with the patient and applicable across all healthcare professionals. Healthcare professionals must realize that knowledge of genetics and epigenetics cannot be isolated from the desired clinical outcome when working with individual patients and must be considered in studies involving populations and communities.

The foundational elements in understanding and utilizing genetic terminology, concepts, and applications are essential if future healthcare professions are to utilize the evolving genetic technologies and must be included in the education for all levels of nurse practitioners and in the scholarship and research activities of nurse educators and practitioners. Technologies for improved testing throughout the life cycle, in the clinic, or at the bedside will advance identifying an individual's genetic makeup and the interaction with the environment.

Pharmacogenetics/Pharmacogenomics and Interprofessional Collaborative Practice Competency Domains

Pharmacogenetics and pharmacogenomics concepts and applications are an excellent foundation in which nurses can collaborate with other healthcare professionals through the four interprofessional collaborative practice competencies developed by IPEC (2011). Nursing—with its focus on optimizing health, preventing disease and illness, alleviating suffering through diagnosis and treatment, and caring for patients and their families as well as in community and population health (Patton, 2006)—is well suited for becoming a key player on the patient-centered team that can contribute or lead the discussion of pharmacogenetics and pharmacogenomics.

The four competencies that apply throughout one's professional education and through one's practice are:

- **Values and Ethics for Interprofessional Practice:** Values and ethics are focused on the patient at the center of the care process by respecting patient dignity and privacy; embracing cultural diversity; respecting roles and responsibilities of others on the healthcare team; developing trusting relationships with patients, families, and other members of the healthcare team; demonstrating high standards of ethical conduct, honesty, and integrity; and maintaining their own professional competency.

- **Roles and Responsibilities:** Healthcare professionals are responsible for communicating their roles to patients, families, and other team members, realizing their limitations when engaging with other healthcare professionals in the care of the patients, communicating effectively to clarify responsibilities, working to develop interdependent relationships, and engaging in professional and interprofessional team development and performance enhancement for optimized patient care.

- **Interprofessional Communication:** Healthcare professionals are effective in various communication techniques leading to organized and effective communication with patients, families, and each other, thus demonstrating the importance of teamwork in patient-centered and community-focused care.
- **Teams and Teamwork:** Promotes and supports other healthcare professionals in shared patient-centered, problem-solving care, which allows for best leadership practices, shared accountability, process improvement strategies, and evidence to inform effective teamwork and team-based practices.

Figure 10.1 shows how nurses who have knowledge and clinical skills in the area of pharmacogenetics and pharmacogenomics are linked to these interprofessional competencies.

In the area of values and ethics, nurses can serve the healthcare team by providing a caring and trusting relationship with a patient, particularly when there are challenging clinical conditions that arise as a function of patients and their families and pharmacogenetic information potentially affecting choices for care. An example would be the conversation with a female patient who has been identified with the BRCA1 gene or the BRCA2 gene associated with a greater risk of developing breast or ovarian cancer. The nurse practitioner (NP) who has developed a trusting and caring relationship would be an excellent representative of the healthcare team to sit and discuss the options that a patient may want to consider to prevent the potential development of breast cancer. A nurse practitioner could also be the individual who helps to manage any ethical dilemmas when there are conflicts between healthcare professionals as to what would be the best option for the treatment plan and the cost-benefit of these treatment options.

With respect to the specific roles and responsibilities, it could be the NP who helps the patient and her family to differentiate and understand the responsibilities of the various healthcare professionals on their teams. The NP could also coordinate the care of the patient as she negotiates between the various healthcare providers in the decision-making process when there are different treatments available from surgery to chemotherapy to radiation based upon genetic cancer markers and findings. The NP can serve as the guide (e.g., patient navigator) through the selected treatment approach to ensure the patient has access to other healthcare professionals who can explain relevant genetic findings.

The NP could also be the one to lead the team in developing continuous professional and interprofessional development in specific areas of expertise ranging from treating genetic-related cancers in specific patient groups (children's leukemia, breast cancer, and prostate cancer).

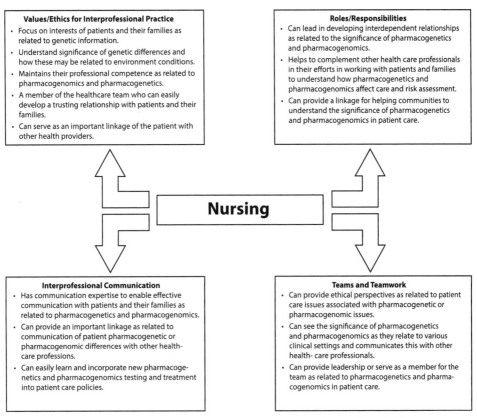

Values/Ethics for Interprofessional Practice
- Focus on interests of patients and their families as related to genetic information.
- Understand significance of genetic differences and how these may be related to environment conditions.
- Maintains their professional competence as related to pharmacogenomics and pharmacogenetics.
- A member of the healthcare team who can easily develop a trusting relationship with patients and their families.
- Can serve as an important linkage of the patient with other health providers.

Roles/Responsibilities
- Can lead in developing interdependent relationships as related to the significance of pharmacogenetics and pharmacogenomics.
- Helps to complement other health care professionals in their efforts in working with patients and families to understand how pharmacogenetics and pharmacogenomics affect care and risk assessment.
- Can provide a linkage for helping communities to understand the significance of pharmacogenetics and pharmacogenomics in patient care.

Nursing

Interprofessional Communication
- Has communication expertise to enable effective communication with patients and their families as related to pharmacogenetics and pharmacogenomics.
- Can provide an important linkage as related to communication of patient pharmacogenetic or pharmacogenomic differences with other health-care professions.
- Can easily learn and incorporate new pharmacogenetics and pharmacogenomics testing and treatment into patient care policies.

Teams and Teamwork
- Can provide ethical perspectives as related to patient care issues associated with pharmacogenetic or pharmacogenomic issues.
- Can see the significance of pharmacogenetics and pharmacogenomics as they relate to various clinical settings and communicates this with other health-care professionals.
- Can provide leadership or serve as a member for the team as related to pharmacogenetics and pharmacogenomics in patient care.

*Based upon Interprofessional Education Collaborative Expert Panel. (2011). Core competencies for interprofessional collaborative practice: *Report of an expert panel.* Washington, D.C.: Interprofessional Education Collaborative.

Figure 10.1   IPEC Core Competencies, Nursing and Pharmacogenetics/ Pharmacogenomics.

Considering interprofessional communications, the NP with effective interprofessional skills could serve as a resource for organizing and providing group presentations for patients and their families, as well as other healthcare professionals, on the topics of new genetic testing methods and their implications for healthcare. An NP with expertise in pharmacogenetics and pharmacogenomics can be the one to develop policies in this area as related to testing and treatments to optimize patient care in an institutional setting. Nurses can also be the individuals who provide timely, constructive feedback to other members of the healthcare team when there are challenging situations, given their expertise in active listening and behavior. Specifically, since they often have direct, daily contact with patients, the nurse could be the individual who has direct communication with the other team members and could share the ideas and opinions provided across the team that are needed for effective decision-making related to specific genetic findings of a given patient.

Nurses can play a key role in educating healthcare professionals and teams in the practices of effective teams and teamwork where pharmacogenetics and pharmacogenomics play an important role in shared patient-centered problem-solving care. Shared patient-centered problem-solving care can be strained in the area of pharmacogenomics/pharmacogenetics, given how quickly new screening technologies and therapies (with increasing costs) are being developed, combined with a lack of consensus on the guiding principles for how the team interacts in these complex healthcare settings. Since nurses are educated as critical health team members in community, long-term, or acute care settings, they can be the bridge that links the outpatient to the long-term care setting or the acute care with the outpatient care setting by taking the leadership role in developing the principles of patient care used across these various teams. An example of this linkage could be in developing the principles in how the plan of a patient's specific healthcare team (such as the acute care situation) is provided to another healthcare team (in the ambulatory setting), particularly when it involves new, genetic-based treatments that might not be as familiar to practitioners in the community setting. The NP can also be the individual who evaluates how well the healthcare team is functioning when involved in the treatment of patients whose cancer diagnosis is associated with a readily identified gene such as the TMPT and leukemia.

There are clearly overlaps in these four core competencies when considering the critical role that nurses can play in providing patient-centered care involving pharmacogenomics and pharmacogenetics. The increasing complexity of pharmacogenetics and pharmacogenomics in patient-centered care will require a team that will be faced with challenges as team members work together to establish their values/ethics for interprofessional practice, identify the roles and responsibilities of team members, decide how they will communicate effectively in current and future interprofessional environments, and examine how the teams and principles of teamwork will need to evolve and develop in the changing healthcare setting. It becomes critical to consider how to optimize inter-professional education for future nursing students at the entry level and graduate level as pharmacogenetics and pharmacogenomics form the foundation for personalized medicine and patient-centered care.

Nursing Students' Pharmacogenetic and Pharmacogenomic Education

The education of future nursing students at all levels must involve the acquisition of knowledge, skills, and attitudes/values in the concepts of pharmacogenetics and pharmacogenomics essential to patient care and in working with other members of the healthcare team. Understanding the interprofessional principles and the four competency domains and the linkage to nursing in the area of pharmacogenetics and pharmacogenomics forms the basis for the education of entry-level nurse practitioners:

- Nurses should know the foundations of genetics and be able to understand key genetic principles and genetic testing technologies so that they can engage effectively in the healthcare team discussions in these areas.

- Nurses must be able to interpret the significance of new genetic findings in the literature as related to clinical care of patients.

- Nurses should promote healthy behaviors (such as healthy eating, exercise, smoking cessation) to minimize risk associated with genetic risk factors associated with the development of cancer, heart disease, or other neurological disorders.

- Nurses need communication skills to work with parents who may be at risk for having children with genetic diseases based upon family history.

- Nurses must be able to use the family history to identify families and individuals who would benefit from genetic testing.

- Nurses must have the knowledge and communication skills to help patients understand results that they may get from commercially available genetic testing options or from tests ordered by their physicians.

Community nurses can play an essential role in providing expertise in pharmacogenetics and pharmacogenomics associated with the patient-centered medical care home models. With early genetic testing in children becoming more common, the nurse can provide another source of information for families and for the healthcare team to understand the significance of the results.

Continuing Professional Development and Graduate Nursing Education in Pharmacogenetics and Pharmacogenomics

With the technologies to be able to sequence the genes for any one individual at an increasingly reduced cost, the need for healthcare professionals with expertise in understanding pharmacogenetic and pharmacogenomic data will be essential as we try to understand how this impacts patient care. Continuing professional development programs must include pharmacogenetics and pharmacogenomics concepts and experiences for those nurses practicing in the variety of evolving healthcare settings. As patients begin to understand their own genetics and its potential impact on their health and wellness, nurses are in an excellent position to work with patients to map out strategies to maximize their health and wellness. For example, if a patient has a gene that would increase risk of cardiovascular disease, a community nurse or nurse in an outpatient setting can help the patient to develop an exercise regimen, stop smoking, change his or her diet, or lose weight, thus reducing the number of factors potentially leading to cardiovascular disease. Graduate nursing education for those pursing an advanced practitioner level or advanced research degree must include courses focusing on the more complex pharmacogenetics and pharmacogenomics principles and opportunities for individuals to have direct, hands-on experiences with these new genetic technologies. Advanced NPs with education in this area can serve as an important resource for applications of clinical care protocols to optimize health, wellness, and patient care in healthcare settings.

For example, the relationships between pharmacogenomics and anesthesia that nurse anesthetists must know is well-established, particularly those related to Cytochrome P-450 enzymes, malignant hyperthermia, and postoperative nausea and vomiting (Ama et al., 2010).

Genetic competencies for advanced nursing degrees were recommended by the American Nursing Association in 2011 (Greco, Tinley, & Seibert, 2012). The areas of professional practice that were recommended include:

- Risk assessment and interpretation

- Genetic education
- Counseling
- Testing and interpretation of test results
- Clinical management of patients
- Ethical, legal, and social implications

Individuals who are doctorally trained in nursing are well positioned to take leadership roles in research that links the increasing genetic information to successful patient outcomes and reduced costs, given their clinical expertise in direct patient care. These nurse researchers whose clinical expertise, including patient observations, assessments, and interpreting clinical data, can combine these findings with the increasing genetic data to investigate for associations that may or may not result in disease or identify effective treatment approaches that can be optimized through knowing patient-specific genetics. Nurse researchers can also utilize large-population genetic data sets in efforts to investigate linkages to disease in specific populations. The opportunities for nurse researchers leading interprofessional research teams focusing on pharmacogenetics and pharmacogenomics will only continue to increase, given the increasing genetic data that will be available at the individual or population level.

Nurses with advanced education would also be expected to provide leadership at the local, state, national, and international level with respect to policies and recommendations. Nurses with advanced clinical and graduate education must play a leadership role in revising the interprofessional core competencies and educational opportunities needed by future practitioners across the health professions.

Summary

The incorporation of new knowledge and skills as related to pharmacogenetics and pharmacogenomics into professional practice requires that current nurses engage in continuous professional development (O'Sullivan, 2006). Continuous professional development in the area of pharmacogenetics and pharmacogenomics requires nurses to recognize the limitations of their knowledge as it relates to genetic terminology and theory, learn technologies for genetic testing and results interpretation, interpret literature findings and applications to clinical care, evaluate ethical and legal issues, and enhance communication skills with other healthcare professionals, patients, and their families.

After the learner identifies the gaps in his or her knowledge and skills, it becomes essential to identify learning activities and desired outcomes needed to address these areas. Lectures and contemporary readings combining active learning activities—such as case studies or direct patient encounters—are essential elements to address these gaps. These types of activities can be coordinated by colleges/schools of nursing through live continuing education programs or hybrids of online learning combined with live small group learning.

Pharmacogenetics and pharmacogenomics learning requires an engaged learner working in a team-based approach to be successful. Furthermore, it requires a culture of learning that is embraced by all members of the healthcare team and by the healthcare organization or setting in which the team works because the field of pharmacogenetics and pharmacogenomics is one where the patient-care technologies will continue to advance with each year.

References

Ama, T., Bounmythavong, S., Blaze, J., Weismann, M., Marienau, M. S., & Nicholson, W. T. (2010). Implications of pharmacogenomics for anesthesia providers. *AANA Journal, 78*(5), 393–399.

American Association of Colleges of Nursing. (2006). The essentials of doctoral education in advanced nursing practice. Washington, D.C. Retrieved from http://www.aacn.nche.edu/dnp/pdf/essentials.pdf

American Association of Colleges of Nursing. (2008). The essentials of baccalaureate education for professional nursing practice. Washington, D.C. Retrieved from http://www.aacn.nche.edu/education/pdf/BaccEssentials08.pdf

American Association of Colleges of Nursing. (2011). The essentials of a master's education in nursing. Draft. Washington, D.C. Retrieved from http://www.aacn.nche.edu/education-resources/MastersEssentials11.pdf

Chial, H. (2008). Rare genetic disorders: Learning about genetic disease through gene mapping, SNPs, and microarray data. *Nature Education 1*(1), 192. Retrieved from http://www.nature.com/scitable/topicpage/rare-genetic-disorders-learning-about-genetic-disease-979

Cronenwett, L., Sherwood, G., Barnsteiner, J., Disch, J., Johnson, J., Mitchell, P., . . . & Warren, J. (2007). Quality and safety education for nurses. *Nursing Outlook, 55*(3), 122–131.

Cronenwett, L., Sherwood, G., Pohl, J., Barnsteiner, J., Moore, S., Sullivan, D., Warren, J. (2009). Quality and safety education for advanced nursing practice. *Nursing Outlook, 57*(6), 338–348.

Greco, K. E., Tinley, S., & Seibert, D. (2012). *Essential genetic and genomic competencies for nurses with graduate degrees.* Silver Spring, MD: American Nurses Association and International Society of Nurses in Genetics.

Interprofessional Education Collaborative Expert Panel (IPEC). (2011). Core competencies for interprofessional collaborative practice: Report of an expert panel. Washington, D.C.: Interprofessional Education Collaborative.

National Research Council. (2003). Health professions education: A bridge to quality. Washington, D.C.: The National Academies Press.

O'Sullivan, J. (2006). Continuing professional development. In R. Jones & F. Jenkins (Eds.) *Developing the allied health care professional* (pp. 1–20). London, UK: Radcliffe Publishing.

Patton, R. M. (2006). Foundations for Practice and Action: Scope and Standards for Practice. *American Nurse Today, 1*(2), 18. Retrieved from http://www.americannursetoday.com/article.aspx?id=5148&fid=5120

The Future of Pharmacogenomics and Nursing

11

Diane Seibert, PhD, ARNP, FAANP, FAAN
Matthew D'Angelo, DNP, CRNA
Michelle Munroe, DNP, CNM

This chapter offers a glimpse of what healthcare might look like when genomics becomes fully integrated into practice. In just two short decades, genomics has evolved from a bench science into an increasingly effective clinical tool. Pharmacogenomics is one area in which genomics is most rapidly becoming clinically useful, having the potential to profoundly change every aspect of healthcare.

Advances in genomic science are revealing genes and biological pathways that influence drug response at the individual patient level. The use of genetic testing to examine the underlying genetic makeup of an individual *prior* to exposing that individual to a drug may make adverse drug reactions (ADRs) outdated, improving both safety and efficacy.

Several topics are described herein to offer readers a glimpse of what future healthcare systems and/or individual health outcomes might look like in a world in which genomics and/or pharmacogenomics are completely integrated into clinical practice.

Genetic Testing Technology

Recent advances in DNA-sequencing technologies have improved to the point that whole genome sequencing (WGS) is now possible

OBJECTIVES

- Whole genome sequencing (WGS) and advances in pharmacogenomics allow for a more personalized approach to healthcare.

- Advances in wearable technology can improve real-time access to healthcare.

- Genomics can increase the effectiveness of a treatment regimen while decreasing the risk for an adverse event.

- Genomic advances are rapidly and profoundly changing healthcare in many (if not all) specialty areas.

for a reasonable price. Within just a few years, WGS may replace the current analyte-based newborn screening process, and the focus will then shift from deciding what tests to order to interpreting existing data. Whenever a new laboratory test is developed, four key concepts must be addressed:

- **Analytic validity:** The degree to which a particular test measures what it is supposed to measure
- **Clinical validity:** Whether the test accurately predicts a particular clinical outcome
- **Clinical utility:** The degree to which a test result influences the treatment plan
- **Personal utility:** The degree to which a result influences an individual's behavior, psychological well-being, and/or clinical outcomes

Many issues are unresolved when these concepts are considered in the context of genetic testing. Analytic validity may soon be largely resolved because genetic testing technologies continue to improve. The establishment of clinical validity for many genetic tests may remain unresolved for years. Currently, clinical validity is clear in monogenic disorders such as cystic fibrosis or Huntington's disease, where specific mutations often reliably predict phenotype. Single gene changes may only account for a 2% to 3% risk increase in highly complex conditions, such as hypertension. It may be many years before the predictive value of traditional risk factors for hypertension—such as obesity, family history, male gender, smoking, and so forth—are surpassed by genomic information.

Clinical utility is available for some conditions now, and more conditions will become actionable in the near future as links between genes and clinical conditions become better understood. Some people have already adopted healthier behaviors or are adhering to preventive therapies based on genomic information, which is likely to increase in the future (Vorderstrasse, Cho, Voils, Orlando, & Ginsburg, 2013).

Electronic Health Records and Family Health Histories

Because genomic healthcare is so heavily dependent on data storage and electronic interpretation, the electronic health record (EHR) is a critical tool because high-speed computing power is needed to help providers make sense of the thousands of gene variants and disorders. In the future, if an individual's entire genome is housed in an EHR, every time a new drug is prescribed, a computer could instantly scan that individual's genome searching for variants that either decrease the efficacy or increase the risk for adverse drug reactions (ADRs) for that particular drug. Although not yet available at the population level, WGS is rapidly declining in cost and may soon replace many of the genetic tests currently being ordered to evaluate an individual's germline genotype. Some of the major questions related to the effective use of EHRs are whether they can efficiently store data, return results rapidly to providers at the point of care, and track outcomes as decision support is adopted.

Family health history (FHH) is a critical piece of data that remains largely ignored by many clinicians because obtaining accurate, complete information at the point of care is such a challenge. Patients often do not know their family medical history. They may keep medical secrets. Families may not share sensitive information, and family members may be adopted or may have died prematurely from nonmedical causes. More robust strategies need to be developed to encourage families to collect and record accurate FHH.

When this information is collected, an EHR should be capable of storing, analyzing, and rapidly retrieving individual genomic information and presenting the raw data along with an interpretation to the clinician at the point of care. An EHR should also be able to link family members in the database, identifying emerging or previously unrecognized health risks or conditions as new data (in the form of diagnosis codes) is entered on individuals in the family. The FHH should be copied forward from one set of individuals (the mother and father) into the child's record to reduce the need to continually collect this information.

New Medications and Patient Responses

Approximately 100 new drug applications are submitted to the U.S. Food and Drug Administration (FDA) annually, making it challenging for clinicians to maintain currency. See the FDA Information on Drugs website (http://www.fda.gov/Drugs/InformationOnDrugs/default.htm) for links to the most up-to-date information on drug shortages, newly approved drugs, and generic equivalent drugs.

Despite the fact that humans are 99.9% similar, there is still an enormous amount of genetic diversity between individuals, even between family members. Although genomic diversity is essential for the survival of any species and is responsible for the wide range of human talents, traits, and characteristics, this diversity presents significant challenges to predicting the way in which an individual will respond to a particular drug. No single medication, therefore, is both safe and effective in everyone.

The debilitating and occasionally deadly consequences of ADRs are associated with high morbidity and mortality and pose significant health, social, and economic burdens for providers, individuals, families, communities, and the healthcare system. Although genetic testing is not routinely used at this time, genomic information can be extremely helpful prior to prescribing drugs associated with severe ADRs in some patients, improving both safety and efficacy.

The FDA Table of Pharmacogenomic Biomarkers lists all the drugs currently on the market that mention pharmacogenomics in their labeling. As of June, 2014, 159 "high risk" drugs were listed in the table. You can view this information at www.fda.gov/drugs/scienceresearch/researchareas/pharmacogenetics/ucm083378.htm

The Potential of Wearable Technologies

Some examples of wearable technologies include wireless wrist trackers, "smart" shirts, and biochips. Incorporation of wireless wearable technology benefits both the wearer and the healthcare provider. It allows the user the ease of a fashionable medical device that provides real-time data that can be remotely accessed by providers.

Wireless Wrist Trackers

Wireless wrist trackers, similar to the fitness trackers currently worn by thousands of people worldwide, could offer many additional features. For example, they might be:

- Built with refillable or replaceable permeable membranes that could deliver medication
- Programmed to vibrate at selected times to remind the wearer to take medications that need to be delivered by other means
- Programmed to monitor several biological parameters

Many healthy people use wireless wristbands to monitor heart rate, activity levels, and sleep to optimize health. Many wireless devices are being used in healthcare settings as well to monitor blood gases, blood glucose, blood pressure, clotting times, drug levels, cardiac function, and to transmit X-ray and ultrasound images. Future applications might include wristbands that constantly monitor drug levels in people at high risk for ADRs due to inherited CYP450 or other metabolism mutations.

"Smart" Shirts

Smart shirts with embedded sensors woven or sewn into them could be programmed to perform many of the functions of the wristbands just described. However, "smart" shirts could be worn by a wider range of people: for example, neonates or young children. Sensors could be woven into other garments as well, such as swimsuits, offering the option of monitoring in wet environments.

Prototypes of wireless shirts are currently being studied in hospitals for respiratory and cardiac disease. As the technology improves, these could be used in infants to decrease the number of deaths in this population from SIDS or respiratory infections (http://portal.uc3m.es/portal/page/portal/actualidad_cientifica/noticias/intelligent_tshirts).

Biochips

Biochips, much like the ID microchips used in pets, could be developed with enough storage capacity that they could store and update financial, demographic, and medical (including genomic) data. The chip could be used as an implantable bank card (reducing the risk of identity theft), could replace passports and medical records, and could be programmed to monitor blood pressure, glucose, and oxygen levels. Biochips could be injected safely and simply into a muscle in the shoulder or hip, using a needle and syringe, much like a vaccine.

Chips would most likely be reserved for emergency use, such as finding lost children, rapidly identifying and locating seriously ill people, increasing the speed and accuracy in an epidemic such as Ebola, or locating victims following a natural disaster, such as Hurricane Katrina. Chips could also provide critical clinical data (Factor V Leiden mutations, CYP450 pathways, and so on) when medical records are unavailable.

There are some significant social and ethical challenges to biochips because they could be implanted without a person's knowledge or consent, and they raise critical issues regarding personal privacy.

Infectious Disease Treatment

New efforts are underway to map the genomes of a large number of common human infectious organisms, such as parasites (malaria and toxoplasmosis), viruses (human, avian, and swine influenza strains; respiratory syncytial virus; rotavirus; West Nile virus; and Eastern equine encephalitis), and bacteria (>1700 strains of klebsiella, acinetobacter, and enterobacter; Dunham, 2014). The hope is that better understanding of the genetic mechanisms of these diverse organisms will allow researchers to develop therapies that circumvent antibiotic resistance, prevent the organisms from evolving enough to jump from one species (such as birds) to humans, and open new pathways to developing vaccines and other therapies.

Rather than waiting for blood culture results to return, which can take 48–72 hours, it may soon be routine to draw a blood sample from a critically ill patient, sequence the genome of the infectious organism, and identify the offending organism at the point of care. Because any antibiotic resistance mutations would be revealed along with the organism's identity, the appropriate therapy could be prescribed immediately. If the patient's genome were already known or were examined simultaneously, the risk for ADRs could also be significantly reduced, particularly important in people who are already critically ill.

Skin and soft tissue infections (SSTIs) are common and have become increasingly antibiotic-resistant, making them difficult to treat. Recent studies exploring the nasal microbiome have found that individuals who did not develop SSTIs had a significantly higher percentage of proteobacteria in their noses than individuals who had resistant SSTIs, suggesting that proteobacteria may protect against the development of SSTIs (USU, 2014). Better understanding of the nasal microbiome may open new prevention strategies targeting the microbiome rather than the infectious organisms.

Obstetrics and Gynecology

The placenta may play a much larger role in the development of complications during the prenatal and intrapartum period than previously thought (Aagaard et al., 2014). Long thought to be sterile, placentas from uncomplicated term pregnancies have recently consistently been found to contain small amounts of DNA from organisms normally found in the mother's oral cavity. In the future, maternal oral samples may provide information about the genetic composition of her microbiome that in turn could provide information about her risks for developing preterm labor, gestational hypertension, and preeclampsia. It may then be possible to identify women at increased risk for adverse pregnancy outcomes, and novel treatment options, such as altering maternal oral microbial environments, might become available to reduce pregnancy complications.

Genetic testing might be used to screen young women for increased susceptibility to the development of gynecologic conditions such as polycystic ovarian syndrome (PCS), infertility, and coagulopathies, which increase the risk of blood clots forming when taking estrogen-containing contraceptives. Testing may also be helpful when providing preconception counseling to identify women at increased risk for neural tube defects who might benefit from higher doses of folic acid. Testing might be used during the perimenopausal period and might identify women who might benefit the most from postmenopausal hormone therapy (HT) based on their genetic risk for severe or prolonged vasomotor symptoms. Finally, genetic testing might also be used to identify women at increased risk for developing ADRs from prolonged exposure to HT.

Neonatal

Newborn screening (NBS) is an area in which dramatic changes are perhaps the closest to being realized. Universal screening for a limited number of treatable conditions that are not usually clinically evident at birth is now offered to all infants born in the United States. Whole genome sequencing (WGS) is still more expensive than NBS, and many questions related to clinical validity and utility still remain unanswered. When the cost for WGS drops below that of NBS, market forces may drive the change from NBS to WGS. When that shift occurs, an individual's entire genome, including information on how she or he is likely to respond to drugs, would be available at or before birth (Fleischer, & Lockwood, 2014). If an infant's entire genome were available for analysis and review, many complicated, time-consuming, and expensive diagnostic workups might be avoided, and the most effective therapies (including pharmacotherapies) could be immediately applied.

Oncology

Germline mutations (present at birth) and somatic mutations (develop over time) are both important in oncology settings because they help to inform diagnosis, prognosis, and treatment. An individual's germline genome can identify individuals at increased risk for developing cancer (BRCA mutations) and determine disease prognosis. However, an individual's germline genome is currently most helpful in calculating an individual's response to drugs, particularly his or her risk for developing ADRs when exposed to a chemotherapeutic agent. The identification and classification of somatic mutations acquired by tumor cells are areas exploding in oncology because the type of mutations a tumor has acquired may predict both the efficacy of a therapeutic intervention or the prognosis if left untreated (Hertz & McLeod, 2013). The integration of germline and somatic genetic information into the development of individualized treatment plans is important because both of these genomic variations are valuable predictors of cancer prognosis and of response and risk for ADRs during exposure to selected chemotherapeutic agents (Mushiroda, Giacomini, & Kubo, 2013).

One emerging area in cancer therapy involves using an individual's own white blood cells (WBCs) to destroy cancer. In this scenario, immediately after the cancer is diagnosed, the individual's blood is drawn and WBCs are filtered and then sorted to identify the WBCs that have developed anticancer antibodies that match the tumor. When grown in the laboratory and infused back into the patient, they could roam throughout the body specifically targeting and killing the cancer cells, potentially eliminating the need to expose the patient to toxic chemotherapy drugs (Tran et al., 2014).

Acute Care Settings

In acute care settings, such as emergency rooms and trauma care units, point of care genetic panel testing could be used to screen patients for CYP450 drug metabolism pathways, rapidly identifying people who may or may not benefit from a particular drug or be at increased risk for ADRs if given a particular drug.

Anticoagulants, often used in acute care settings, are considered "high risk" drugs because too much medication increases the risk for hemorrhage (stroke, gastrointestinal bleeding), while too little medication can cause dangerous clotting events (stroke, myocardial infarction, pulmonary embolus). Point of care genotyping platforms have already been developed and deployed for two high-risk anticoagulants: clopidogrel (Plavix) and warfarin (Coumadin), which provide a good example for what might be possible for many medications in the future.

Clopidogrel (Plavix) is an anticoagulant commonly used in acute care settings in combination with aspirin to help prevent blood clots that may cause a heart attack or stroke. The CYP2C19 gene is responsible for producing an enzyme that is needed to transform clopidogrel into its active form. At least eight versions of CYP2C19 have been identified, altering the metabolism rates of drugs that are metabolized by the CYP2C19 pathway. These alterations in drug metabolism help to explain why clopidogrel doesn't inhibit clotting to the same extent in everyone who is prescribed it, and why these individuals are at increased risk for heart attacks, strokes, and sudden death, despite being on the drug.

Warfarin (Coumadin) is an anticoagulant that prevents new blood clots from forming and/or prevents existing blood clots from worsening. A dosing table has been added to the warfarin label providing suggested dose ranges based on genotype (VKORC1, CYP2C9*2 and *3). The clinical benefit of genetic testing is still unclear; the Clinical Pharmacogenetics Implementation Consortium (CPIC) recommends genotype-based dosing. Other groups, such as the American College of Chest Physicians, recommended against routine genetic testing because evidence from randomized control trials has not shown a clinical benefit. In the future, as more information on how genetic testing impacts health outcomes becomes available, point-of-care testing for many drugs and metabolic pathways may become a routine part of care.

Pain and Rehabilitation

Opioids are widely used in pain management, but the amount of pain relief and risk for significant ADRs varies dramatically between individuals, even between members of the same family. Optimizing drug selection and dose can be challenging because some people metabolize opioids rapidly and do not receive full therapeutic benefit, whereas others experience unpleasant or dangerous side effects because the drugs persist longer than expected in circulation. Genetic testing for variations in CYP450 pathways (CYP2D6 and CYP2C19, in particular) help to explain much of the variability in opioid response, and genetic testing (or review of WGS data) may become standard of care prior to prescribing any pain medications to increase the efficacy and decrease ADRs in patients who need pain medication.

In addition to screening people for drug metabolism pathways, genetic testing may someday be used to reveal genes associated with an increased risk for developing pain, such as fibromyalgia, migraine headaches, osteoarthritis, endometriosis, Crohn's disease, temporomandibular disorder, and others. People found to be at increased genetic risk for developing migraine headaches, for example, might be counseled in childhood to avoid headache triggers, such as fluorescent light, perfume, smoking, skipping meals, alcohol, and tyramine-containing foods (Goadsby & Silberstein, 2013).

The management of acute injury and rehabilitation is likely to change. Additionally, the genes associated with inflammation and sepsis will become better understood. Researchers are already exploring the possibility of using gene-expression techniques in critically ill patients to profile neutrophils and reliably diagnose sepsis from other noninfectious conditions. This work is likely to reveal insights into the host response to sepsis (Tang, McLean, Dawes, Huang, & Lin, 2007). These and similar findings may help classify the variety of sepsis presentations into subcategories that can then be managed through more appropriate fluid resuscitation or pharmacologic treatment.

Genes associated with collagen formation, skin integrity, constipation, falls, and so on might be used to identify people at increased risk for adverse outcomes while simultaneously guiding treatment planning in sports medicine, rehabilitation, or long-term care facilities.

Obesity

Many human body functions are regulated by human genes alone, yet function in concert with the genes of the thousands of microbes that live in and on the human body: the "human microbiome." Obesity researchers are actively exploring the relationships and interactions between the human genome and the human microbiome because the microbiome has been shown to be both protective and synergistic. The human microbiome protects the body from a hostile takeover from more lethal microorganisms; produces essential nutrients; and plays major roles in digestion, nutrient absorption, and immune regulation (Grice & Segre, 2012). Microorganisms begin colonizing the skin and gastrointestinal (GI) tract at (and perhaps prior to) birth, and the quantity and type of organisms shift over a lifetime in response to dietary changes, geographic location, age, medications (particularly antibiotics), and stress (Bäckhed et al., 2012).

Recent studies have shown that certain types and members of microbial families are associated with obesity. Obese adults have more firmicutes and fewer bacteroidetes species than leaner adults. However, as overweight adults lose weight, the balance shifts, with bacteroidetes colonies increasing and birmicutes colonies declining with weight loss (Cani et al., 2012; Ley, Turnbaugh, Klein, & Gordon, 2006). In the future, strategies for helping people lose weight may include the collection of a fecal sample, which could be tested to determine what type of GI flora that individual has, and an individualized drug cocktail might be developed specifically for that person to help them lose weight or maintain weight loss.

Gut flora also appear to be involved in regulation of host immunity. The development of irritable bowel disease (IBD), such as colitis and Crohn's disease, has been associated with the pattern of GI microbes a person has acquired (Li et al., 2012). *B. infantis,* for example, has been shown to simultaneously reduce GI inflammation while suppressing proinflammatory cytokines such as interferon-gamma (IFN-γ), tumor necrosis factor-alpha (TNF-α), and IL-12 (Konieczna, Akdis, Quigley, Shanahan, & O'Mahony, 2012). Probiotics such as lactobacilli, bifidobacteria, and nonpathogenic yeasts such as *Saccharomyces boulardii,* have been shown to support immune function, decrease inflammation, and prevent weight gain (Poutahidis et al., 2013). In the future, deliberate manipulation of the types or numbers of bacteria using antibiotics, probiotics, exercise, or special diets may all become important therapeutic options in managing inflammatory GI disorders and reducing obesity (Baumler, 2013; Herman, 2014).

Summary

Changes are happening rapidly at both the bench and the bedside, and it is a challenge for all healthcare professionals to remain informed as new information emerges into practice. Nurses must remain alert for new information that affects their practice and make adjustments to practice as disease screening and management recommendations change with the emergence of new research findings. This chapter offers just a brief glimpse of how the future of healthcare might look as genomics is infused into everyday practice.

Questions

Clinical utility is:

   a. The degree to which a particular test measures what it is supposed to measure

   b. Whether the test accurately predicts a particular clinical outcome

   c. The degree to which a test result influences the treatment plan *

   d. The degree to which that result influences an individual's behavior, psychological well-being, and/or clinical outcomes

The electronic health record (EHR) will be a critical tool as genomics continues to infuse into healthcare for all the following reasons except:

   a. High-speed computing power can help providers make sense of the thousands of gene variants and disorders.

   b. EHRs can archive, organize, and display salient FHH information when it is needed at the point of care.

   c. When WGS becomes widely used, EMRs will be needed to store and present the data.

   d. The EHR could reliably predict which family member will develop a particular disorder. *

Nasal proteobacteria:

   a. May protect against the development of Crohn's disease

   b. May protect against the development of SSTIs *

   c. May protect against the development of obesity

   d. May protect against the development of chronic pain

Placentas from uncomplicated term pregnancies have recently been found to contain small amounts of DNA from organisms normally found in:

   a. The mother's oral cavity *

   b. The mother's rectum

   c. The mother's nasal passages

   d. The mother's vagina

Somatic mutations:

   a. Are present at birth

   b. Develop over time *

   c. Are associated only with cancers

   d. Are entirely responsible for cancer development

References

Aagaard, K., Ma, J., Antony, K. M., Ganu, R., Petrosino, J., & Versalovic, J. (2014). The placenta harbors a unique microbiome. *Science Translational Medicine, 6*(237), 237ra65.

Bäckhed, F., Fraser, C. M., Ringel, Y., Sanders, M. E., Sartor, R. B., Sherman, P. M., … Finlay, B. B. (2012). Defining a healthy human gut microbiome: Current concepts, future directions, and clinical applications. *Cell Host & Microbe, 12*(5), 611–622. doi:10.1016/j.chom.2012.10.012

Baumler, M. D. (2013), Gut bacteria. *Today's Dietitian, 15*(6), 46.

Cani, P. D., Osto, M., Geurts, L., & Everard, A. (2012). Involvement of gut microbiota in the development of low-grade inflammation and type 2 diabetes associated with obesity. *Gut Microbes, 3*(4), 279–288. doi:10.4161/gmic.19625

Clarke, S. F., Murphy, E. F., O'Sullivan, O., Lucey, A. J., Humphreys, M., Hogan, A., . . . Cotter, P. D. (2014). Exercise and associated dietary extremes impact on gut microbial diversity. *Gut.* Advance online publication. doi: 10.1136/gutjnl-2013-306541.

Dunham, W. (2014). U.S. backs new genetic research on infectious diseases. *Reuters Health Information.* Retrieved from http://www.reuters.com/article/2014/06/05/us-usa-health-grant-idUSKBN0E-G2PM20140605

Fleischer, J. A., & Lockwood, C. M. (2014). Newborn screening by Whole-Genome Sequencing: Ready for prime time? *Clinical Chemistry, 60*(9), 1243-1244.

Goadsby, P. J., & Silberstein, S. D. (2013). Migraine triggers: Harnessing the messages of clinical practice. *Neurology, 80*(5), 424–425.

Grice, E. A., & Segre, J. A. (2012). The human microbiome: Our second genome. *Annual Review of Genomics and Human Genetics, 13*(1), 151–170. doi:10.1146/annurev-genom-090711-163814

Hertz, D. L., & McLeod, H. L. (2013). Use of pharmacogenetics for predicting cancer prognosis and treatment exposure, response and toxicity. *Journal of Human Genetics, 58*(6), 346–352.

Konieczna, P., Akdis, C. A., Quigley, E. M., Shanahan, F., & O'Mahony, L. (2012). Portrait of an immunoregulatory Bifidobacterium. *Gut Microbes, 3,* 261–266.

Ley, R. E., Turnbaugh, P. J., Klein, S., & Gordon, J. I. (2006). Human gut microbes associated with obesity. *Nature, 444*(21), 1022–1023. doi:10.1038/nature4441022a

Li, E., Hamm, C. M., Gulati, A. S., Sartor, B., Chen, H., Wu, X., . . . Frank, D. (2012). Inflammatory bowel diseases phenotype, C. difficile and NOD2 genotype are associated with shifts in human ileum associated microbial composition. *PLoS One, 7:*e26284.

Mushiroda, T., Giacomini, K. M., & Kubo, M. (2013). Special section on pharmacogenomics: Recent advances and future directions. *Journal of Human Genetics, 58*(6), 305.

Poutahidis, T., Kleinewietfeld, M., Smillie, C., Levkovich, T., Perrotta, A., Bhela, S., . . . Erdman, S. E. (2013). Microbial reprogramming inhibits Western diet-associated obesity. *PLoS One, 8*(7), e68596. doi:10.1371/journal.pone.0068596

Tang, B. M., McLean, A. S., Dawes, I. W., Huang, S. J., & Lin, R. C. (2007). The use of gene-expression profiling to identify candidate genes in human sepsis. *American Journal of Respiratory and Critical Care Medicine, 176*(7), 676–684.

Tran, E., Turcotte, S., Gros, A., Robbins, P. F., Lu, Y. C., Dudley, M. E., . . . Rosenberg, S. A. (2014). Cancer immunotherapy based on mutation-specific CD4+ T cells in a patient with epithelial cancer. *Science, 344*(6184), 641-645.

Uniformed Services University of the Health Sciences (USU). (2014, May 21). Nasal bacteria may be predictor of skin infections. ScienceDaily. Retrieved from www.sciencedaily.com/releases/2014/05/140521094318.htm

Vorderstrasse, A. A., Cho, A., Voils, C .I., Orlando, L. A., & Ginsburg, G. S. (2013). Clinical utility of genetic risk testing in primary care: The example of type 2 diabetes. *Personalized Medicine, 10*(6), 549–563.

Numbers

Index

A

B

D

E

Q–R